The Children's Pharmacy

The Children's Pharmacy

EVERYTHING YOU SHOULD KNOW ABOUT MEDICINES FOR YOUR CHILDREN

By

ANNE CAREY, R.N.

THE BOBBS-MERRILL COMPANY, INC.
Indianapolis/New York

Published by The Bobbs-Merrill Company, Inc.
Indianapolis/New York
Manufactured in the United States of America
First Printing
Designed by Jacques Chazaud

Library of Congress Cataloging in Publication Data

Carey, Anne.
    The children's pharmacy.

    Includes index.
    1. Drugs—Popular works. 2. Pediatric pharmacology.
I. Title.
RJ560.C27   1983   615.5'42   84-20712
ISBN 0-672-52727-8

CAUTION:

This book is not intended, nor should it be regarded, as medical advice. Before giving your child any drug, prescription or over-the-counter, consult your doctor. It is your doctor's function to diagnose your child's medical problem and prescribe the appropriate medicine, dosage, and course of therapy.

Special thanks to:

Ross S. Laderman, Director, Consumer and Professional Staff, U.S. Food and Drug Administration, for his generous assistance and skillful guidance; and to Mark Hunter for his inestimable help in the preparation of this book. Also to Dr. Martin Feldman, who reviewed and approved the book for accuracy.

Contents

Introduction

By Martin Feldman, M.D.

It is important that parents be aware of *all* of the effects of the drugs they are giving to their children. In *The Children's Pharmacy*, you will find facts about the drugs most commonly prescribed for your children. Arranged according to the disease or problem for which they are prescribed. Anne Carey's comprehensive book provides an excellent vehicle for parents to exercise caution in giving medicine to their children. With no prior medical knowledge, the parents can have at their fingertips easy and immediate access to the relevent data pertaining to the drug they are giving their child. This book is a superb guideline for concerned parents who want to use discretion in choosing their children's medications.

Know Your Enemy
During the growing years, a child's body is biochemically sensitive. Drugs taken during these years can affect the natural growth processes. It is unfortunately true that we are giving our youth a large quantity of prescribed drugs. The potential adverse reactions of each drug described in this book will help you in making qualified decisions as to the specific drug your child should be taking.

Most of the medications given to children do not treat the medical problem but a symptom of the problem. Constantly eliminating the symptom only pacifies the underlying problem and leads to reoccurring illness. Many ailments will subside within a few days without the use of medicine. Also, many times a symptom may indicate that the body is healing itself. For example, the body increases in temperature while in the process of destroying bacteria.

Over-the-counter drugs should be used with caution, as they, too, can produce serious side effects. Administering medication does not always result in the best health for the child. The long-term effect of continued drug usage can be just the opposite.

I urge you to read Chapter 13 first. "A Rapid Guide to Miscellaneous Prescription Drugs for Children" and its corresponding code are invaluable in determining if the drug prescribed should be given to your child. This guide instructs you as to when *not* to give your child a specific drug. It is imperative that you know if your child is included in the cautionary categories pertaining to a certain medication. This guide is an absolute must for every household with children.

Less Is Better

Most of the drugs prescribed for children are for minor ailments such as a cold, flu, or fever. There are some diseases such as diabetes, heart disease, and some digestive ailments, of course, in which medication is mandatory. For lesser illnesses, however, a child should be given medication only when absolutely necessary. The side effects of continual drug use can outweigh its benefits in the child's overall health. Prescription and over-the-counter drugs should not be consistently used to treat symptoms. When necessary, the medicine needed should be used only for a brief period. In these cases, it is advisable to administer the least possible dosage, medically monitor the child while using the medication, and stop the medication as soon as possible. Time-release tablets often result in an increased dosage, as well as prolonging any adverse reactions that might occur. Combinations of different drugs can also prove to be dangerous and should be avoided.

The Alternative?

Insisting on a prescription drug to remedy your child's temporary illness will be detrimental to the health in the long run. Many times the body can and will simply heal itself. We need to teach our children to take care of their bodies properly, both in prevention and in times of illness. Natural healing can often take place without drugs but instead with the help of vitamins and diet. Vitamins, minerals, a healthy diet, fresh air, and exercise should not be underestimated. For cold and flu problems, vitamin A, vitamin C, and calcium are often helpful. In some cases, psychological counseling is beneficial in disease prevention. Frequent infections are a common cause for prescribing medication. However, if the body is given a chance to fight these infections, it builds a stronger immune system. Non-drug alternatives to combatting infection are easily accessible in the form of vitamin A, zinc, and vitamin C.

Shaping Our Children's Attitudes

As a child who is consistently given medication is more likely to become a drug-dependent adult, parents need to consider seriously their responsibility as role models for their children. Our society uses drugs indiscriminately, with the least excuse, or with no reason whatsoever. Drugs, both legal and illegal, are characteristic of our culture. As parents, we remedy any problem with a pill. This example has undoubtedly contributed to the drug-oriented culture we have today. Parents need to begin to teach their children that drugs used correctly equals drugs used sparingly. In alerting parents as to the variety and severity of the side effects of children's prescription drugs, *The Children's Pharmacy* will help to produce a new generation of drug-free children and adults.

How to Use
This Book

The purpose of this book is to provide you with reliable and understandable information about therapeutic drugs for your children. As an informed consumer, you will be better equipped to work together with your doctor and pharmacist to provide for your children's health.

In this book you'll find a representative selection of prescription (℞) and over-the-counter (OTC) drugs that, according to manufacturers' claims, are useful in the treatment of children's disorders. Of those drugs, those most commonly prescribed are preceded by a check mark (√).

To locate drugs for the treatment of specific diseases, refer to the Contents or the Index. To locate specific drugs, refer to the Index. To find the characteristics of a drug belonging to a drug family, refer to the description of that drug family. That description is supplied under the following headings:

Trade name or names

Ingredients

These drugs are used to

How these drugs work

The FDA has
    ☐ Approved these drugs.
    ☐ Not approved these drugs.

These drugs are
    ☐ Effective.
    ☐ Probably effective.
    ☐ Ineffective.

These drugs should not be used under the following conditions

Your doctor may not approve use of these drugs under the following conditions

Use of the following drugs decreases the effectiveness of these drugs

How these drugs interact with other drugs

How these drugs are supplied

Dosage

Common side effects

Effect or effects of long-term use

After-use effect or effects

Information is supplied in the same manner for some drugs which are not members of drug families. Information on other drugs in that category is capsulized.

Because of the complexity of drug regulations, some drugs not acceptable to the Food and Drug Administration (FDA) are legally marketable. The FDA bases its acceptance on safety and effectiveness. Should your children's doctor prescribe a drug not approved by the FDA, ask for an explanation, or write for information to: Director, Consumer and Professional Staff, U.S. Food and Drug Administration, Bureau of Drugs, HFD-5, 5600 Fishers Lane, Rockville, MD 20857. Follow the same procedure if your doctor prescribes a drug characterized by the FDA as "probably effective."

1

Drugs to Treat Emotional Disorders

DRUGS TO TREAT ATTENTION-DEFICIENCY DISORDERS (HYPERACTIVITY)

I. NONPHENOTHIAZINES

Trade name
   √ CYCLERT (℞).

Ingredient
   Pemoline, a member of a family of drugs called central stimulants.

This drug is used to
   Treat attention-deficiency disorders in children, characterized by hyperactivity, short span of attention, inability to sit still, excitability, lack of concentration, impulsiveness (usually prolonged), and ease with which the child is distracted. Attention-deficiency disorders were formerly

known as MBD, minimal brain dysfunction. This drug is prescribed for children 6 years of age or over.

How this drug works
The exact mechanism has not been established.

The FDA has
☑ Approved this drug.
☐ Not approved this drug.

This drug is
☑ Effective.*
☐ Probably effective.
☐ Ineffective.

This drug should not be used under the following condition
• Sensitivity to Pemoline.

Your doctor may not approve use of this drug under the following condition
• Kidney or liver disorders.

Use of the following drug decreases the effectiveness of this drug
No drugs with this action reported.

How this drug interacts with other drugs
No significant reactions reported.

How this drug is supplied
Tablets, chewable tablets.

*But maximum effectiveness may not be achieved for several weeks.

Dosage

37.5 mg. per day, 4 times a day, first dose in the morning; increased weekly by 18.75 mg. per day to a maximum 112.5 mg. or until desired results occur. Maintenance dose: 56.25 to 75 mg. per day.

Common side effects

Insomnia, loss of appetite, loss of weight, dizziness, drowsiness, nausea, stomach ache, headache, irritability, depression, skin rash. *Warning:* Diminished alertness may occur; should it, be sure your child does not engage in any potentially hazardous activity requiring alertness.

Effects of long-term use

Cyclert may cause retroperitoneal fibrosis and changes in liver function. Possibility of physical and/or psychological dependence. Other long-term effects not established.

After-use effects

Withdrawal symptoms can be avoided by gradual dosage reduction.

Trade name
    √ *RITALIN* (℞).

Ingredient
    Methylphenidate hydrochloride, a member of a family of drugs called central stimulants.

This drug is used to
    Treat attention-deficiency disorders in children characterized by hyperactivity, short span of attention, inability to sit still, excitability, lack of concentration, impulsiveness (usually prolonged), and ease with which the child is distracted. Attention-deficiency disorders were formerly known as MBD, minimal brain dysfunction. This drug is prescribed for children 6 years of age or over and is also used to treat mild depression and narcolepsy (sudden attacks of sleep or irresistible desire to sleep during normal waking hours).

How this drug works
    The exact mechanism has not been established.

The FDA has
        ☑ Approved this drug.
        ☐ Not approved this drug.

This drug is
        ☑ Effective.*
        ☐ Probably effective.
        ☐ Ineffective.

This drug should not be used under the following conditions
    • Sensitivity to methylphenidate hydrochloride.

*But only probably effective when used to treat mild depression.

24

- Severe depression, anxiety, tension, or agitation.
- Glaucoma.
- Epilepsy.

Your doctor may not approve use of this drug under the following condition
- High blood pressure.

Use of the following drugs decreases the effectiveness of this drug
No drugs with this action reported.

How this drug interacts with other drugs
- Decreases the blood-pressure-lowering effect of guanethidine.
- Adverse reactions are possible when this drug is used simultaneously with certain medicines for "thinning blood" (coumarin-type anticoagulants) and for treating depression (tricyclic antidepressants and MAO inhibitors); with a medicine to treat certain types of joint disease (phenylbutazone); and with medicines to treat seizures, asthma, and other breathing problems.

How this drug is supplied
Tablets.

Dosage
5 mg. each before breakfast and lunch. May be increased weekly by 5 to 10 mg. per day to a maximum of 60 mg.

Common side effects
Insomnia, loss of appetite, nausea, stomach ache, headache, dizziness, drowsiness. *Warning:* Diminished alertness may occur; should it, be sure your child does not

engage in any potentially hazardous activity requiring alertness.

Effects of long-term use
Possibility of psychological dependence and weight loss. Overall effects of long-term use not known.

After-use effects
Your doctor may terminate use of this drug by decreasing dosage gradually to prevent possible withdrawal symptoms.

II. PHENOTHIAZINES

Trade names
See page 30.

Ingredients
Chlorpromazine and chlorpromazine hydrochloride.

These drugs are used to
Treat attention-deficiency disorders (hyperactivity) in disturbed and mentally retarded children, usually on a short-term basis. For a description of these disorders, see pages 21-22 under this head. These drugs are also used to treat psychotic agitation, aggressiveness, and explosive, intense excitability.

How these drugs work
It is likely that these drugs interfere with a chemical reaction in the brain and curtail the release of certain hormones.

The FDA has
    ☑ Approved these drugs.
    ☐ Not approved these drugs.

These drugs are
☑ Effective.*
☐ Probably effective.
☐ Ineffective.

These drugs should not be used under the following conditions
• Sensitivity to phenothiazines.
• Impaired function of the bone marrow, particularly decreased red cell production (bone marrow depression).
• Reyes syndrome (an acute illness of childhood characterized by fever, vomiting, disturbance of consciousness progressing to coma, and convulsions).

Your doctor may not approve use of these drugs under the following conditions
• Heart disease.
• Blood or blood vessel disease.
• Liver disease.
• Lung disease.
• Difficulty in urinating.
• Severe asthma, emphysema, or acute respiratory disease.
• Epilepsy.

Use of the following drugs decreases the effectiveness of these drugs
Antimuscarinics (drugs which restrain some actions of the involuntary nervous system, such as dilation of the blood vessels).

*But most effective in treatment of psychiatric disorders characterized by psychotic agitation, aggressiveness, and explosive, intense excitability.

How these drugs interact with other drugs
- Act like barbiturates on CNS depressants, including barbiturates. See page 35.
- These drugs interact with other drugs less likely to be prescribed for children. Inform your doctor of all drugs your child is taking. While your child is on these drugs, do not give the child any other drug, prescription or nonprescription, without the approval of your doctor.

How these drugs are supplied
See under individual drugs, page 30.

Dosage
See under individual drugs, page 30.

Common side effects
Restlessness; excitement; shuffling walk; trembling; shaking hands and fingers; jerky movements of head and neck; involuntary tongue and mouth movements; fast heartbeat; stuffed nose; dry mouth; decreased sweating; increased sensitivity of the skin to sunlight; skin rashes; difficulty urinating; muscle spasms in the neck, back, and other parts of the body; weight gain; diminished sex drive; changes in menstrual period; breast swelling; light-headedness; fainting; dizziness; drowsiness. *Warning:* Should drowsiness occur, be sure your child does not engage in any potentially hazardous activity requiring alertness. There are many other adverse reactions which are less likely to occur, such as fever, jaundice (a liver disease characterized by a yellowing of the skin), and bone marrow depression (a reduction in the ability to manufacture blood cells). Check with your doctor at once should your child show any side effect.

Effects of long-term use
   Consult your doctor.

After-use effects
   Sudden withdrawal may produce side effects which can be avoided by gradual reduction of dosage.

The drugs
   Chlorpromazine products which may be prescribed for children are listed alphabetically by product name. The ingredient for each product is listed as well as other pertinent information not covered in the preceding general description.

√ *CHLORPROMAZINE HYDROCHLORIDE (HCL)* (℞). See THORAZINE.

MELLARIL (℞). Tablets, concentrate. Thioridazine hydrochloride. This drug is used to treat children whose excessive hyperactivity is accompanied by misconduct. Dosage: 10 mg. 2 to 4 times a day to start, unless symptoms are severe, in which case starting dose is 25 mg. 2 to 4 times a day. Dosage can be increased to a maximum of 3 mg. per kilogram (about 2.2 lb.) of body weight per day.

MELLARIL-S (℞). Oral suspension. Thioridazine. See MELLARIL.

√ *THORAZINE* (℞). Tablets, capsules, syrup, concentrate, rectal suppositories, ampules, and vials. Chlorpromazine hydrochloride. Also used to treat pre- and postoperative anxiety, and nausea and vomiting. Dosage (only for treatment of hyperactivity): orally .25 mg. per pound of body weight, daily every 4 to 6 hours as needed; parenterally (by injection), .25 mg. per pound of body weight intramuscularly every 6 to 8 hours daily as needed. For other uses of Thorazine, see page 45.

DRUGS TO TREAT ANXIETY AND OTHER EMOTIONAL DISORDERS

I. ANTIHISTAMINES

Trade names
See under specific drugs beginning on page 33.

Ingredients
Hydroxyzine hydrochloride or hydroxyzine pamoate, both antihistamines.

These drugs are used to
Treat anxiety, an abnormal emotional state character-ized by a fear that something terrible is going to happen, despite no real basis for that fear. Anxiety often manifests itself in physical symptoms such as breathlessness, abnormal breathing, muscular constriction, pain in the chest (as well as elsewhere), fast pulse, belching, diarrhea or constipation, indigestion, and fatigue. Sometimes the physical symptoms are unaccompanied by fear. These drugs are also used to treat emotional disturbances, stress, and agitation. *Warning:* Parents must give careful consideration to a child's symp-toms in order to distinguish normal childhood fears from serious emotional disturbances. Though the symptoms of anxiety can be temporarily quieted with drugs, nondrug

therapies (psychiatric or psychological counseling) may offer the only "cure."

How these drugs work
They act on the central nervous system to produce a sedative effect.

The FDA has
☑ Approved these drugs.
☐ Not approved these drugs.

These drugs are
☑ Effective.
☐ Possibly effective.
☐ Ineffective.

These drugs should not be used under the following condition
• Sensitivity to hydroxyzine.

Your doctor may not approve use of these drugs under the following condition
Consult your doctor.

Use of the following drugs decreases the effectiveness of these drugs
No drugs with this action reported.

How these drugs interact with other drugs
• Act like bariturates on CNS depressants. See page 225.

How these drugs are supplied
Tablets, capsules, oral suspensions (liquid), and syrup.

Dosage

By mouth: for children under 6 years of age: 50 mg. per day, divided doses; for children over 6 years of age: 50 to 100 mg. a day, divided doses. By intramuscular injection, .6 mg. per kilogram (about 2.2 lb.) of body weight in a single dose.

Common side effects

Dryness of mouth and daytime drowsiness. *Warning:* Should daytime drowsiness occur, be sure your child does not engage in any potentially hazardous activity requiring alertness.

Effects of long-term use

None reported.

After-use effects

None reported.

The drugs

Antihistamines which may be prescribed for children are listed alphabetically by product name. The ingredient for each product is listed as well as other pertinent information not covered in the preceding general description. When no ingredient is listed, the name of the drug is the sole ingredient.

√ *ATARAX* (℞). Tablets, syrup. Hydroxyzine hydrochloride.

√ *HYDROXYZINE HYDROCHLORIDE INJECTION* (℞). Vials.

√ *HYDROXYZINE HCL, USP* in Tubex (℞), a closed injection system which delivers this drug in accurately machine-measured doses. Available in 25, 50, and 100 mg. units.

√ *HYDROXYZINE HYDROCHLORIDE TABLETS* (℞). Available in 10, 25, and 50 mg. tablets.

√ *VISTARIL* (℞). Hydroxyzine pamoate. Capsules, oral suspension. This drug is also used to treat anxiety related to organic disease; other nervous and emotional conditions; anxiety before surgery and after anesthesia; and some forms of skin itch.

II. BARBITURATES

Trade names
   See page 37.

Ingredients
   See under specific drugs, beginning on page 37.

These drugs are used to
   Treat anxiety. (For a description of anxiety, see page 31.)

How these drugs work
   They depress the central nervous system. These drugs also have sedative and sleep-inducing properties.

The FDA has
   ☑ Approved these drugs.
   ☐ Not approved these drugs.

These drugs are
   ☑ Effective.
   ☐ Probably effective.
   ☐ Ineffective.

These drugs should not be used under the following conditions
   See page 224.

Your doctor may not approve use of these drugs under the following conditions
See page 225.

The use of the following drugs decreases the effectiveness of these drugs
See page 225.

How these drugs interact with other drugs
See page 225.

How these drugs are supplied
Elixir, tablets.

Dosage
See under individual drugs, beginning on page 37.

Common side effects
See page 226. *Warning:* Alertness may be decreased, should this occur, prevent children from engaging in potentially hazardous activities requiring alertness.

Effect of long-term use
Possibly addictive.

After-use effects
Consult your doctor.

The drugs
Barbiturates which may be prescribed for children are listed alphabetically by product name. The ingredient of each product is given as well as dosage and other pertinent information not covered in the preceding general description.

√ *BUTICAPS* (℞). Capsules. Sodium butabarbital. Dosage for daytime sedation: 7.5 to 30 mg.

√ *BUTISOL SODIUM* (℞). Elixir. See BUTICAPS.

NEMBUTAL (℞). Elixir. Pentobarbital. Dosage for daytime sedation depends on age, weight, and condition, as determined by your doctor.

NEMBUTAL SODIUM (℞). See NEMBUTAL.

√ *PHENOBARBITAL* (℞). Capsules, drops, elixir. Phenobarbital. Oral dosage for daytime sedation: 6 mg. per kilogram (about 2.2 lb.) of body weight per day in 3 divided doses; parenteral (injected) dosage: 8 to 30 mg., intramuscularly.

√ *PHENOBARBITAL SODIUM* (℞). Ampules, vials, syringes, cartridge-needle units. Phenobarbital sodium. See PHENO-BARBITAL.

SECONAL (℞). See page 228.

SECONAL SODIUM (℞). See page 228.

√ *S-K PHENOBARBITAL* (℞). Tablets. See PHENOBARBITAL.

√ *SOLFOTON* (℞). See page 228.

III. BENZODIAZEPINES

Trade names
      See page 40.

Ingredients
      See under specific drugs, beginning on page 40.

These drugs are used to
      Treat anxiety. (For a description of anxiety, see page 31.) For other uses of these drugs, see under drugs on page 40.

How these drugs work
      They act on sections of the nervous system.

The FDA has
            ☑ Approved these drugs.
            ☐ Not approved these drugs.

These drugs are
            ☑ Effective.*
            ☐ Probably effective.
            ☐ Ineffective.

*Bensodiazepines may be the most effective and safest of the anti-anxiety drugs.

*These drugs should not be used under the following
condition*
- Sensitivity to ingredients.

*Your doctor may not approve use of these drugs under the
following conditions*
- Hyperactivity (attention-deficiency disorders).
- Depression.
- Severe chronic obstructive pulmonary diseases.
- Kidney and liver disorders.
- Epilepsy.
- History of drug abuse or dependence.
- Psychotic behavior.
- Myasthenia gravis (chronic, progressive weakness of
  the voluntary muscles).

*Use of the following drugs decreases the effectiveness of
these drugs*
No drug with this action reported.

How these drugs interact with other drugs
- Act like barbiturates on CNS depressants, including
  barbiturates. See page 225.

How these drugs are supplied
Capsules, ampules, tablets.

Dosage
See under individual drugs, page 40.

Common side effects
Mental confusion, blurred vision, dryness of mouth,
unsteadiness, constipation, difficulty urinating, dizziness,
light-headedness, headache, nausea, fatigue, drowsiness.

Warning: Should signs of drowsiness occur, be sure your child does not engage in any potentially hazardous activity requiring alertness.

Effects of long time use
    None reported.

After-use effects
    Sudden withdrawal effects may include trouble sleeping, anxiety, irritability, nervousness, sweating, trembling, nausea or vomiting, stomach and/or muscle cramps, confusion, and nightmares.

The drugs

CHLORDIAZEPOXIDE HCL (R). Capsules. See LIBRIUM.

√ *LIBRAX* (R). Capsules. Chlordiazepoxide hydrochloride (a benzodiazepine) and clidinium bromide. Used mainly to treat painful stomach and intestinal spasms. As a mild tranquilizer, it treats anxiety associated with that disorder. Dosage: No general guidelines have been established. Do not use if child has an obstruction at neck of bladder.

LIBRITABS (R). Tablets. See LIBRIUM.

LIBRIUM (R). Capsules, ampules. Chlordiazepoxide hydrochloride. Used to treat mild to acute and preoperative anxiety. Dosage: For children over 6 years of age, 5 mg. 2 to 4 times daily. Parenteral (injectable) form is not prescribed for children under 12. Do not use in case of glaucoma, shock, or comatose state.

SK-LYGEN (R). Capsules. See LIBRIUM.

IV. MEPROBAMATES

Trade names
    See page 43.

Ingredient
    Meprobamate.

These drugs are used to
    Treat anxiety. (For a description of anxiety, see page 31.) These drugs are also used to relieve nervousness and tension, and for sedation.

How these drugs work
    They act on several areas of the central nervous system. he exact mechanism is not known.

The FDA has
        ☑ Approved these drugs.
        ☐ Not approved these drugs.

These drugs are
        ☑ Effective.*
        ☐ Probably effective.
        ☐ Ineffective.

*But not as effective as benzodiazepines.

These drugs should not be used under the following conditions
- Sensitivity to meprobamate and related drugs.
- Porphyria (a congenital metabolic disorder that causes abnormalities in nerve and muscle tissue).

Your doctor may not approve use of these drugs under the following conditions
- Epilepsy.
- Liver or kidney disorders.

Use of the following drugs decreases the effectiveness of these drugs
No drugs with this action reported.

How these drugs interact with other drugs
- Act like barbiturates on CNS depressants, including barbiturates. See page 225.

How these drugs are supplied
Capsules, tablets.

Dosage
100 to 200 mg. 2 to 4 times a day for children 6 to 12 years of age.

Common side effects
Unsteadiness; blurred vision; change in vision; slurred speech; headache; nausea; vomiting; fatigue; diarrhea; skin rash; hives; itching; feeling "high"; dizziness; sensation of burning, pricking, or numbness; daytime drowsiness. *Warning:* Should signs of drowsiness occur, be sure your child does not engage in any potentially hazardous activity requiring alertness.

Effects of long-term use
    Possibility of addiction.

After-use effects
    Withdrawal symptoms may include trouble sleeping, nightmares, more dreams than usual, irritability, nervousness, restlessness, unsteadiness, mental confusion, twitching, trembling, convulsions, or seizures.

The drugs
    Meprobamates which may be prescribed for children are listed alphabetically by product name. Pertinent information not covered in the preceding general description is given.

EQUANIL (R). Capsules.

MEPRIAM (R). Tablets.

MEPROBAMATE (R). Tablets.

MEPROSPAN (R). Capsules, controlled release.

MILTOWN (R). Tablets. Do not use Miltown 600.

SK-RAMATE (R). Tablets.

V. PHENOTHIAZINES

Trade names
    See below and page 45.

Ingredients
    Members of the phenothiazine family of drugs. For ingredients of individual drugs, see under drugs below and on page 45.

These drugs are used to
    Treat anxiety and other emotional disorders. For other uses, see under individual drugs below and on page 45.
    For a profile of phenothiazines, see page 54. For dosage, see under individual drugs in the following list.

The drugs
    Phenothiazines which may be prescribed for children are listed alphabetically by product name. The ingredient for each product is listed as well as other pertinent information not covered in the preceding general description.

STELAZINE. (R) Tablets, concentrate, vials. Trifluoperazine hydrochloride. For the treatment of excessive anxiety. Dosage: For hospitalized children 6 to 12 years of age, 1 mg. 2 to 4 times a day, raised to up to 15 mg. This drug is also used for the treatment of psychotic disorders.

THORAZINE. (℞) Tablets, capsules, syrup, concentrate, rectal suppositories, ampules, and vials. Chlorpromazine hydrochloride. Used to treat pre- and postoperative anxiety. Dosages for children over 6 months of age: oral dosage, preoperative, .25 mg. per pound of body weight, 2 to 3 hours prior to surgery; postoperative, .25 mg. per pound every 4 to 6 hours, as needed. Parenteral (injection) dosage: preoperative, .25 mg. per pound of body weight injected intramuscularly 1 hour to 2 hours prior to surgery, postoperative, .25 mg. per pound, repeated in 1 hour if needed. This drug is also used to treat psychic disorders and intense nausea and vomiting.

DRUGS TO TREAT
PSYCHOTIC DISORDERS

Trade names
   Thorazine and similar drugs.

Ingredients
   Members of the phenothiazine family of drugs. See references under drugs below.
   For a profile of phenothiazines, see page 27.

The drugs

COMPAZINE. (℞) Tablets, capsules (controlled-release), syrup, concentrate, ampules, vials, syringe, suppositories. Prochlorperazine. Used to treat psychiatric conditions in children. Oral dosage for children 2 to 12 years of age: 2.5 mg. 2 to 4 times a day; 10 mg. maximum on day 1; can be increased to 20 mg. per day for children 2 to 5 years of age and to 25 mg. per day for children 6 to 12 years of age, as needed. Parenteral (injected) dosage: .06 mg. per pound of body weight injected intramuscularly for children under 12 years of age.

MELLARIL (℞). See page 30.

STELAZINE (℞). See page 44.

√ *THORAZINE* (℞). See page 45.

DRUGS FOR SEDATION

Trade names
See list of drugs below.

Ingredients
See under individual drugs below.

How these drugs work
Act to calm nervous excitement.
For profiles of drugs for sedation, turn to pages indicated in the following list.

The drugs

√ *ATARAX* (℞). See page 50.

√ *BUTICAPS* (℞). See page 37.

√ *BUTISOL SODIUM* (℞). See page 37.

√ *DALMANE* (℞). See page 229.

√ *NOCTEC* (℞). See page 232.

√ *PHENOBARBITAL* (℞). See page 227.

√ *THORAZINE* (℞). See page 55.

2

Drugs to Treat Motion Sickness, Nausea, and Vomiting

DRUGS TO TREAT MOTION SICKNESS

I. ANTIHISTAMINES

Trade names
    See list of drugs in this section.

These drugs are used to
    Treat motion sickness, which may be triggered by any kind of travel, and is characterized by nausea, retching, and vomiting. Other possible symptoms are fatigue prior to nausea, clammy skin, dizziness, disorientation (not knowing where you are), and blurred vision. Motion sickness may be triggered when travel motions overstimulate the semicircular canals in the ears. Nausea and vomiting can result from causes other than travel motion. Though antihistamines are regarded by many physicians as the drugs of

choice in the treatment of motion sickness, they have many other uses.

How these drugs work

The exact mechanism is unknown, but it is likely that these drugs counter overstimulation of the semicircular canals of the ears, act on the central nervous system, and interfere with a chemical (acetylcholine) which helps transmit messages along the nervous system.

For a profile of antihistamines, see page 31.

For dosages, see individual drugs in the following list.

The drugs

Antihistamines which may be prescribed for children are listed alphabetically by product name. The ingredient for each product is listed as well as pertinent information not covered in the general description on page 31.

√ *ANTIVERT* (℞). Tablets, chewable tablets. Meclizine hydrochloride. Dosage: for children 12 years of age and over, 25 to 50 mg. 1 hour prior to travel; repeat every 24 hours, as needed. *Warning:* Antivert should be used with caution—or not at all—in the treatment of children.

√ *ATARAX* (℞). Tablets, syrup. Hydroxyzine hydrochloride. Your doctor will determine dosage depending on age, weight, and condition. See page 33.

√ *BENADRYL* (℞). Capsules, elixir. Diphenhydramine hydrochloride. Dosage for children over 20 pounds, 12.5 to 25 mg. 3 to 4 times a day, taken 30 minutes prior to travel, before meals, and at bedtime while traveling.

√ *BONINE* (OTC). Chewable tablets of 25 mg. each. See ANTIVERT.

√ *DIMENHYDRINATE* (OTC). Tablets. See DRAMAMINE, below.

DIPHENHYDRAMINE HYDROCHLORIDE (OTC). Capsules, elixir, injectables. See BENADRYL, page 50.

√ *DRAMAMINE* (OTC). Capsules, liquid. Dimenhydrinate. Dosage: for children 2 to 6 years of age, 12.5 to 25 mg. every 4 to 6 hours, up to 75 mg. in 24 hours; for children 6 to 12 years of age, 25 to 50 mg. every 6 to 8 hours, up to 150 mg. in 24 hours.

√ *MAREZINE* (OTC). Tablets. Cyclizine hydrochloride. Dosage: for children 12 years of age and older, 1 tablet (50 mg.) 1/2 hour prior to travel; repeat every 4 to 6 hours as needed; 4 tablets maximum. For children 6 to 12 years of age, 1/2 tablet up to 3 times a day.

√ *VISTARIL* (℞). Tablets, syrup. See ATARAX, page 50.

II. A NONANTIHISTAMINE

Trade name
      √ *EMETROL* (OTC).

Ingredients
      Fructose, glucose, and orthophosphoric acid in balanced amounts, mint-flavored.

This drug is used to
      Relieve the nausea and vomiting of motion sickness. This drug also relieves vomiting from other causes, and regurgitation in infants.

How this drug works
      It provides fast relief by acting directly on the wall of the gastrointestinal (GI) tract to reduce muscular contraction.

The FDA has
            ☑ Not disapproved this drug.
            ☐ Disapproved this drug.

This drug is
            ☑ Effective.
            ☐ Probably effective
            ☐ Ineffective.

This drug should not be used under the following conditions
   None reported.

Your doctor may not approve use of this drug under the following conditions
   None reported.

Use of the following drugs decreases the effectiveness of this drug
   None reported.

How this drug interacts with other drugs
   No adverse reactions reported.

How this drug is supplied
   Oral solution.

Dosage
   1 teaspoon for young children, 1 tablespoon for older children. Do not dilute. Prevent your child from drinking other liquids from 15 minutes before to 15 minutes after taking this drug.

Common side effects
   No adverse side effects reported.

Effects of long-term use
   No adverse effects reported.

After-use effects
   No adverse effects reported.

DRUGS TO TREAT NAUSEA AND VOMITING NOT ASSOCIATED WITH MOTION SICKNESS

I. PHENOTHIAZINES

Trade names
See list of drugs in this section.

These drugs are used to
Treat nausea and vomiting usually associated with anesthesia, surgery, cancer therapy, cancer, and kidney failure. They are also used to treat psychoses.

How theses drugs work
They have a sedative or tranquilizing effect on the central nervous system and inhibit the vomiting impulse.
For a profile of phenothiazines, see page 44.
For dosages, see individual drugs in the following list.

The drugs
Phenothiazines which may be prescribed for children are listed alphabetically by product name. The ingredient for each product is listed as well as pertinent information not covered in the general description on page 44.

√ *CHLORPROMAZINE HYDROCHLORIDE* (℞). Tablets, capsules, syrup, concentrate, injectables. See THORAZINE.

√ *COMPAZINE* (℞). Tablets, capsules (sustained-released), syrup, concentrate, ampules, vials, syringe, rectal suppositories. Prochlorperazine. For severe nausea and vomiting. Dosage: for children 20 to 29 lb., 2.5 mg. 2 to 3 times a day (or up to 7.5 mg. a day); for children 30 to 39 lb., 2.5 mg. 2 to 3 times a day (or up to 10 mg. a day); for children 40 to 85 lb., 2.5 mg. 3 times a day, or 5 mg. 2 times a day (or up to 15 mg. a day).

√ *PHENARGIN* (℞). Tablets, syrup, rectal suppositories. Promethazine hydrochloride. Dosage is determined by your doctor based on child's age, weight, and condition.

√ *PROCHLORPERAZINE TABLETS* (℞). See COMPAZINE.

√ *PROMETHAZINE HYDROCHLORIDE (HCL)* (℞). Tablets, syrup, injectables. See PHENARGIN.

√ *THORAZINE* (℞). Tablets, capsules (sustained-release), syrup, concentrate, ampules, vials, rectal suppositories. Chlorpromazine hydrochloride. Dosage: for nausea and vomiting in children over 6 months of age, oral dosage is .25 mg. per pound of body weight every 4 to 6 hours; parenteral (injected) dosage for children 6 months to 5 years old, or less than 50 pounds, .25 mg. per pound intramuscularly every 6 to 8 hours, up to 75 mg. per day if required. For nausea and vomiting during surgery, no oral dosage permitted; parenteral dosage for children over 6 months of age, .125 mg. per pound of body weight injected intramuscularly and repeated in ½ hour if required; consult your doctor about alternate dosage. Your doctor will monitor blood pressure, since this drug may produce a sharp drop in blood pressure.

VESPRIN (℞). Tablets, suspension, vials, syringe. Triflupromazine hydrochloride. For severe nausea and vomiting. Oral dosage for children 2½ to 12 years of age: .2 mg. for every kilogram (about 2.2 lb.) of body weight, in 3 divided doses daily up to 10 mg. per day. Parenteral (injected) dosage for children 2½ to 12 years of age: .2 to .25 mg. for every kilogram (about 2.2 lb.) per day, up to 10 mg. per day.

II. NONPHENOTHIAZINES

Trade names
    Barbiturate products.
    Some doctors prescribe some barbiturates to treat nausea and vomiting. For a profile of barbiturates, see page 35.

Trade name
    √ *PEPTO-BISMOL* (OTC).

Ingredients
    Bismuth subsalicylate.

This drug is used to
    Treat indigestion and diarrhea.

The FDA has
    ☑ Not disapproved this drug.
    ☐ Not approved this drug.

This drug is
    ☑ Effective.
    ☐ Probably effective.
    ☐ Ineffective.

This drug should not be used under the following conditions
    • When diarrhea is accompanied by a high fever (101.5 degrees or higher).
    • When diarrhea continues for two days while on this drug.
    Caution: In both of the preceding cases, contact your doctor at once.

Your doctor may not approve use of this drug under the following conditions
    None reported, except for drug interactions.

Use of the following drugs decreases the effectiveness of this drug
    None reported.

How this drug interacts with other drugs
- Drugs containing salicylate or acetominophen should be monitored if child is also taking aspirin or drugs labeled acetaminophen. Toxicity could result. Increases the side effects of aspirin. Discontinue use of Pepto-Bismol should ringing in the ears occur.
- Adverse effects may result from taking this drug in combination with medicines for thinning blood, diabetes, or gout.

How this drug is supplied
Liquid, tablets.

Dosage
Liquid dosage for children 3 to 6 years of age, ½ teaspoon; 6 to 10 years of age, 1 teaspoon; dosage repeated every ½ to 1 hour as needed. Maximum dosage: 8 teaspoons.

Common side effects
Temporary darkening of the stools and tongue.

Effects of long-term use
Long-term use is not indicated.

After-use effects
No adverse effects reported.

Trade name
    √ *TIGAN* (℞).

Ingredient
    Trimethobenzamide hydrochloride. The pediatric suppository also contains benzocaine.

This drug is used to
    Treat nausea and vomiting, particularly in cases where cause of vomiting is known.

How this drug works
    The exact mechanism is not established, but this drug may act on that area in the brain controlling the vomiting impulse.

The FDA has
        ☑ Approved this drug
        ☐ Not approved this drug

This drug is
        ☑ Effective.*
        ☐ Probably effective.
        ☐ Ineffective.

This drug should not be used under the following conditions
    • Sensitivity to trimethobenzamide.
    • Sensitivity to benzocaine when suppository is used.

Your doctor may not approve this drug under the following conditions
    • High fever.

*One side effect may be continued severe vomiting.

- Intestinal infection
- Reye's syndrome (see page 28).

Use of the following drugs decreases the effectiveness of this drug
None reported.

How this drug interacts with other drugs
- Acts like barbiturates on CNS depressants, including barbiturates. See page 225.

How this drug is supplied
Capsules, pediatric suppositories.

Dosage
Oral dosage for children 30 to 90 pounds: 100 to 200 mg. 3 to 4 times a day. Rectal suppository dosage for children under 30 lb., 100 mg. 3 or 4 times a day; for children 30 to 90 lb., 100 to 200 mg. 3 to 4 times a day.

Common side effects
Blurred vision, headache, back pain, muscle cramps, dizziness, mental depression, sore throat, fever, fatigue, diarrhea, shaking, seizures, yellow eyes and skin, continued severe vomiting, drowsiness. *Warning:* Should signs of drowsiness occur, prevent your child from engaging in any potentially hazardous activity requiring alertness.

Effects of long-term use
No adverse effects reported.

After-use effects
No adverse effects reported.

Trade name
   WANS Children (Webcon Anti-Nausea Supprettes)
(℞).

Ingredients
   Pyrilamine maleate, an antihistamine, and phenobarbital sodium, a barbiturate.

This drug is used to
   Treat prolonged vomiting the cause of which is known.

How this drug works
   Pyrilamine maleate is a type of antihistamine (an ethylenediamine) which acts to relieve nausea and vomiting. Phenobarbital sodium, a general CNS depressant, acts on the vomiting center and provides sedation.
   For a profile of antihistamines, see page 31; and of barbiturates, page 35.

The FDA has
   ☐ Approved this drug.
   ☑ Not approved this drug.

This drug should not be used under the following conditions
   • Sensitivity to antihistamines or barbiturates.
   • Barbiturate addiction.
   • Severe liver disorders.
   • Uncontrolled pain.
   • Head injury associated with vomiting or other CNS (central nervous system) disturbances.
   • Acute intermittent porphyria (see page 42).

Your doctor may not approve use of this drug under the following conditions
   • Any previous or present drug dependence.
   • Hyperactivity.

- Psychological disturbances.
- Suicidal tendencies.
- Severe anemia.
- Congestive heart failure.
- Hyperthyroidism.
- Fever.
- Diabetes.
- Asthma.
- Chronic lung diseases.
- Liver or kidney disorders.
- Stomach ulcer.
- High blood pressure.
- Intestinal blockage.
- Urinary tract blockage.
- Underactive adrenals.

Use of the following drugs decreases the effectiveness of this drug
    None reported.

How this drug interacts with other drugs
- Acts like barbiturates on CNS depressants, including barbiturates. See page 225.
- Interferes with the action of blood thinners (anti-coagulants), corticosteroids, cardiac glycosides, and numerous other drugs. Inform your doctor of all drugs, prescription and nonprescription, your child is taking; and do not give the child any additional drug without your doctor's approval.

How this drug is supplied
    Pediatric rectal suppositories.

Dosage
    Dosage for children 2 to 12 years of age or weighing over 15 kg. (about 33 pounds): 1 suppository every 6 to 8

hours daily as needed, up to 3 suppositories every 24 hours. For children 6 months to 2 years of age, or under 15 kg., ½ dosage indicated in preceding sentence. *Caution:* Overdosage can result in severe illness.

Common side effects
Headache; blurred vision; slurred speech; increased sweating; faster heartbeat; diarrhea; difficulty urinating; pains in joints and muscles; dry mouth, nose, and throat; hangover; dizziness; light-headedness; unsteadiness; drowsiness. *Warning:* Should signs of drowsiness occur, deter your child from engaging in any potentially hazardous activity requiring alertness.

Effect of long-term use
May be addictive.

After-use effects
Trouble in sleeping, increased frequency of dreams, nightmares, hallucinations, restlessness, weakness, faintness, trembling.

3

Drugs to Treat the Common Cold and the Flu

Trade names
See the list of drugs in this section, page 66.

Ingredients
See under individual drugs in this section, page 66.

These drugs are used to
Relieve the symptoms of the common cold and the flu. There is no cure for the common cold. Some vaccines may provide immunity to certain strains of viruses causing flu. The major symptoms of the common cold and the flu are sore throat, runny nose, sneezing, coughing, watery eyes, nasal congestion, sinus pressure, sinus congestion, headache, body aches and pains, fever, and postnasal drip. Severe colds and flu are characterized by symptoms which include coughing, fever, and body aches and pains, which may be absent in common colds.

How these drugs work
This is what the classes of drugs in cold/flu medicines do:
   • *Analgesics*—act to reduce the sensibility to pain.

- *Anesthetics*—act to produce partial or complete loss of sensation.
- *Antibacterials*—act to destroy bacteria. In cold/flu medicines, they act to counter secondary bacterial infections.
- *Anticholinergics*—act to reduce mucus flow, drying up runny and clogged nasal and sinus passages.
- *Antihistamines*—act to reduce mucus flow, runny nose, and sneezing.
- *Antipyretics*—act to reduce fever.
- *Antitussives*—act to relieve coughing.
- *Decongestants*—act to shrink swollen tissues in the nose, sinuses, and throat.
- *Expectorants*—act to help loosen mucus deposits in the breathing passages.
- *Stimulants*—act to elevate mood and provide a feeling of well-being.

The FDA has
    ☑ Approved these drugs.*
    ☐ Not approved these drugs.

The drugs

√ *ACTIFED-C EXPECTORANT* (℞). Syrup. For the relief of coughing. Triprolidine hydrochloride (antihistamine), pseudoephedrine hydrochloride (decongestant), codeine phosphate (antitussive), guaifenesin (expectorant). Reacts like barbiturates on CNS depressants, including barbiturates (see page 225), and decreases the effectiveness of certain blood-pressure-control medicines. Do not use if child is

Warning: Drugs containing salicylate or acetaminophen should be closely monitored if a child is also receiving drugs labeled as aspirin or acetaminophen. Toxicity could result. See also under individual drugs in this section and warning concerning aspirin, page 152.

sensitive to any ingredient, or has asthma or any lower-respiratory-tract disease. Your doctor may not prescribe this drug if child has high blood pressure or heart or thyroid disease. Dosage for children 12 years of age and over, 2 teaspoons 3 to 4 times daily; for children 6 to 12 years of age, 1 teaspoon; for children 4 to 6 years of age, ¾ teaspoon; and for children 2 to 4 years of age, ½ teaspoon. Dosage should be individualized according to the needs and response of the child. Common side effects include mild stimulation and sedation (in younger children; the stimulation occurs more often than sedation); dizziness; clumsiness; and dryness of nose, mouth, and throat. May be addictive. For the relief of cough in the common cold (and other conditions), the FDA has classified this drug as "lacking substantial evidence of effectiveness as a fixed combination."

AMBENYL-D (OTC). Decongestant cough formula. Liquid. Guaifenesin (expectorant), pseudoephedrine hydrochloride (decongestant), dextromethorphan hydrobromide (antitussive). Do not use if child is sensitive to any ingredients, or has high blood pressure, heart disease, diabetes, or thyroid disease. Should your child show no improvement within 7 days, or rash, or a headache that won't go away, consult your doctor before proceeding further with this medicine. Reacts adversely with antidepressant drugs containing a MAO (monoamine oxidase) inhibitor and with prescription drugs for hypertension (high blood pressure). Dosage for children 6 to 12 years of age, 1 teaspoon every 6 hours; 2 to 6 years of age, ½ teaspoon every 6 hours.

√ AMBENYL EXPECTORANT (℞). Liquid. For the relief of cough in the common cold. Codeine sulfate (antitussive), bromodiphenhydramine hydrochloride (antihistamine), diphenhydramine hydrochloride (antihistamine and anti-tussive), ammonium chloride (expectorant), potassium guaiacolsulfonate (expectorant), menthol (coolant), and alcohol (sedative and solvent). Reacts like barbiturates on CNS depressants, including barbiturates (see page 225). Do not use if child is sensitive to any of the ingredients or has asthmatic attacks, narrow-angle glaucoma, peptic ulcer, or bladder-neck or pyloroduodenal obstruction. Your doctor may not prescribe this drug if your child has a history of asthma. Dosage for children 6 to 12 years of age, ½ to 1 teaspoon every 6 hours; for children 2 to under 6 years of age, ¼ to ½ teaspoon every 6 hours. Common side effects include confusion; nervousness; restlessness; nausea; vom-iting; diarrhea; blurring of vision and double vision; diffi-culty urinating; constipation; palpitations; sensitivity to light; anemia; low blood pressure; tingling sensation; dry-ness of mouth, nose, and throat; drowsiness. *Warning:* Should signs of drowsiness occur, deter your child from engaging in any potentially hazardous activity requiring alertness. This drug may be addictive. For the control of cough in the common cold (or allergy), the FDA has classi-fied this drug as follows: "There is a lack of substantial evidence that this fixed combination drug has the effect purported."

√ *ANACIN* (OTC). Tablets, capsules. Aspirin (analgesic, anti-pyretic) and caffeine (stimulant). For a profile of aspirin, see page 151. Dosage for children 6 to 12 years of age, 1 tablet or capsule every 4 hours as needed, but not more than 5 doses in 24 hours unless more are prescribed by a doctor.

BAYER ASPIRIN (OTC). Tablets. For relief of painful dis-comfort and fever of colds, flu, and other disorders. For a profile of aspirin (analgesic, antipyretic), see page 151. Dos-age for children over 12 years of age, 1 to 2 tablets with water every 4 hours, up to 12 tablets a day; for children under 12 years of age, the following dosages, which may be repeated every 4 hours, but not more than 5 times a day: 11 to under 12 years of age, 1½ tablets; 9 to under 11 years of age, 1¼ tablets; 6 to under 9 years of age, 1 tablet; 4 to under 6 years of age, ¾ tablet; 2 to under 4 years of age, ½ tablet; under 2 years of age, consult your doctor.

√ *BAYER CHILDREN'S CHEWABLE ASPIRIN* (OTC). Orange-flavored tablets. See BAYER ASPIRIN in this section. Dosages, which may be repeated every 4 hours, but not more than 5 times a day: for children 12 years of age or over (84 lb. or over of body weight), 8 tablets; for children 11 to 12 years of age (77 to 83 lb. of body weight), 6 tablets; for children 9 to 11 years of age (66 to 76 lb. of body weight), 5 tablets; for children 6 to 9 years of age (46 to 65 lb. of body weight), 4 tablets; for children 4 to 6 years of age (36 to 45 lb. of body weight), 3 tablets; for children 2 to 4 years of age (27 to 35 lb. of body weight), 2 tablets; for children under 2 years of age, consult your doctor.

√ *BAYER CHILDREN'S COLD TABLETS* (OTC). Orange-flavored chewable tablets. To relieve nasal congestion, ease breathing, reduce fever, and relieve minor aches and pains of cold and flu. Phenylpropanolamine hydrochloride (decongestant), aspirin (analgesic/antipyretic). Your doctor may not approve use of this drug if your child has asthma, diabetes, thyroid or heart disease, or high blood pressure. Dosages, which may be repeated every 4 hours but not more than 4 times a day: for children 6 to 12 years of age, 4 tablets; for children 4 to 5 years of age, 2 tablets; for children 3 to 4 years of age, 1 tablet, for children under 3 years of age, consult your doctor. Common side effects are sleeplessness, nervousness, and dizziness.

√ *BAYER COUGH SYRUP FOR CHILDREN* (OTC). Cherry-flavored. Phenylpropanolamine hydrochloride (decongestant), dextromethorphan hydrobromide (antitussive). Your doctor may not approve the use of this drug if your child has asthma, diabetes, thyroid or heart disease, or high blood pressure. Dosage for children 6 to 12 years of age, 2 teaspoons every 4 hours, up to 8 in 24 hours; for children 2 to 5 years of age, 1 teaspoon every 4 hours, up to 4 teaspoons in 24 hours; for children under 2 years of age, consult your doctor.

BAYER TIMED-RELEASE ASPIRIN (OTC). Tablets. See BAYER ASPIRIN in this section. Dosage for children over 12 years of age, 1 tablet every 8 hours, 2 before bedtime, up to 6 tablets in 24 hours; for children under 12 years of age, consult your doctor.

√ *BENYLIN COUGH SYRUP* (OTC). Raspberry-flavored. Diphenhydramine hydrochloride (antihistamine), alcohol (sedative and solvent). For a profile of antihistamines, see page 31. Do not use without consulting your doctor if your child has epilepsy, glaucoma, difficulty urinating, high blood pressure, heart or thyroid disorders, or if your child is sensitive to this drug. Should the cough persist after 7 days, or should your child exhibit a high fever, rash, or a headache that won't go away, consult your doctor. Dosage for children 6 to 12 years of age, 1 teaspoon every 4 hours, up to 6 teaspoons in 24 hours; for children 2 to under 6 years of age, ½ teaspoon every 4 hours, up to 3 teaspoons in 24 hours; for children under 2 years of age, consult your doctor.

BENYLIN DM (OTC). Cough syrup, imitation-raspberry flavored. Dextromethorphan hydrobromide (antitussive), alcohol (sedative, solvent). Reacts adversely with antidepressive drugs containing a MAO (monoamine oxidase) inhibitor. Your doctor may not approve the use of this drug if your child has asthma or a liver disorder. Dosage for children 6 to 12 years of age, ½ to 1 teaspoon every 4 hours, or 1½ teaspoons every 6 to 8 hours, up to 6 teaspoons in 24 hours; for children 2 to under 6 years of age, ¼ to ½ teaspoon every 4 hours, or ¾ teaspoon every 6 to 8 hours, up to 3 teaspoons in 24 hours; for children under 2 years of age, consult your doctor.

√ *CHILDREN'S CoTYLENOL LIQUID COLD FORMULA* (OTC). Cherry-flavored. Used to relieve all symptoms of common cold and flu except redness and swelling. Acetaminophen (analgesic, antipyretic), chlorpheniramine maleate (antihistamine), phenylpropanolamine hydrochloride (decongestant). Do not use this drug if your child is sensitive to any of its ingredients or is taking a prescription drug for high blood pressure or emotional disorders. Do not use without consulting your doctor if your child has asthma, glaucoma, high blood pressure, heart disease, diabetes, or thyroid disease. Should symptoms fail to improve in 7 days, or should your child exhibit a high fever or persistent cough, consult your doctor. Dosage for children 11 years of age, 3 teaspoons every 4 hours as needed, up to 4 doses in 24 hours; for children 9 to 10 years of age, 2½ teaspoons; for children 6 to 8 years of age, 2 teaspoons; for children 4 to 5 years of age, 1½ teaspoon; for children 2 to 4 years of age, 1 teaspoon. Common side effects are nervousness, restlessness, and sleeplessness.

√ *CHILDREN'S TYLENOL* (OTC). Chewable tablets, elixir, drops. Relieves fever and painful discomfort of the common cold and the flu. Acetaminophen (analgesic, antipyretic). Dosages may be repeated 4 or 5 times daily, up to 5 doses in 24 hours. For the chewable tablets: children 11 to

12 years of age, 6 tablets; 9 to 10 years of age, 5 tablets; 6 to 8 years of age, 4 tablets, 1 year to 2 years of age, 1½ tablets. For the elixir: children 11 to 12 years of age, 3 teaspoons; 9 to 10 years of age, 2½ teaspoons; 6 to 8 years of age, 2 teaspoons; 4 to 5 years of age, 2.4 ml.; 2 to 3 years of age, 1.6 ml.; 12 to 23 months, 1.2 ml.; 4 to 11 months, .8 ml.; birth to 3 months, .4 ml. This drug, according to the manufacturer, "has rarely been found to produce any side effects."

√ *CODEINE* (℞).* Liquid, tablets, injectables. For relief of pain, troublesome cough. Codeine is the generic name. It is an antitussive and an analgesic. Codeine compounds appear in many cold/flu medicines. It reacts like barbiturates on CNS depressants, including barbiturates (see page 35) and reacts adversely with medicines for stomach cramps or spasms. Dosage, for pain relief, .5 mg. per kilogram (about 2.2 lb.) of body weight, 4 to 6 times a day; for cough relief in children 6 to 12 years of age, 5 to 10 mg. every 4 to 6 hours, up to 60 mg. a day. Common side effects include constipation, nausea, vomiting, feeling of excitement, breathing difficulties, slow heartbeat, dizziness, light-headedness, fainting, drowsiness. *Warning:* Should signs of drowsiness occur, deter your child from engaging in any potentially hazardous activity which requires alertness. May be addictive.

√ *CONGESPIRIN* (OTC). Chewable cold tablets for children. For the temporary relief of fever, pain, nasal congestion, runny nose, and sneezing from cold or flu. Aspirin (analgesic, antipyretic) and phenylephrine hydrochloride (decongestant). For a profile of aspirin, see page 151. Your doctor may not approve use of this drug if your child has high fever, high blood pressure, diabetes, or heart or thy-

*In compounds approved by your doctor.

roid disease. Dosage, which may be repeated every 4 hours, up to 4 doses a day: for children 12 years of age or over, 8 tablets; for children 11 years of age, 6 tablets; for children 9 to 10 years of age, 5 tablets; for children 6 to 8 years of age, 4 tablets; for children 4 to 5 years of age, 3 tablets; for children 2 to 3 years of age, 2 tablets; for children under 2 years of age, consult your doctor. Do not use for more than 10 days without the approval of your doctor.

√ *CONGESPIRIN LIQUID COLD MEDICINE* (OTC). In addition to action of Congespirin chewable cold tablets for children (see preceding entry), this drug reduces swelling of the nasal passages, restoring freer breathing. Acetaminophen (analgesic, antipyretic), phenylpropanolamine hydrochloride (decongestant). Your doctor may not approve use of this drug if your child has high fever, high blood pressure, diabetes, or heart or thyroid disease. Dosage, which may be repeated up to 4 times a day, for children 6 to 12 years of age, 2 teaspoons every 3 to 4 hours; for children 3 to 5 years of age, 1 teaspoon every 3 to 4 hours; for children under 3 years of age, consult your doctor. Do not use for more than 10 days without the approval of your doctor.

CONTAC Continuous Action Decongestant Capsules (OTC). Provides up to 12 hours of prolonged relief from nasal congestion due to the common cold (and other sources). Pheynlpropanolamine hydrochloride (decongestant) and chlorpheniramine maleate (antihistamine). For a profile of antihistamines, see page 49. Do not use if your child has high blood pressure, glaucoma, diabetes, asthma, heart or thyroid disease, or if your child is taking another medicine containing phenylpropanolamine. Dosage for children 12 years of age or older, 1 capsule every 12 hours; for dosage for children ,under 12 years of age, consult your doctor. Common side effects are dizziness, sleeplessness, nervousness, drowsiness. *Warning:* Should signs of drowsiness occur, deter your child from engaging in any potentially hazardous activity requiring alertness.

√ *CONTAC JR. The Complete Cold Medicine for Children* (OTC). Liquid. Relieves all cold symptoms. Phenylpropanolamine hydrochloride (decongestant), acetaminophen (analgesic, antipyretic), dextromethorphan hydrobromide (antitussive), alcohol (sedative and solvent). Do not use if your child is taking another medicine containing phenylpropanolamine hydrochloride. If your child has a high fever, severe or recurrent pain, diabetes, or heart disease, consult your doctor before using this drug. Also consult your doctor if symptoms persist after 7 days of use. Dosage: Follow instructions on label, but consult your doctor concerning dosage for children under 31 pounds or under 3 years of age. The manufacturer does not report any common side effects.

CONTAC Severe Cold Formula (OTC). Capsules. Treats colds with flulike symptoms. Pseudoephedrine hydrochloride (decongestant), acetaminophen (analgesic, antipyretic), dextromethorphan hydrobromide (antitussive), chlorpheniramine maleate (antihistamine). For a profile of antihistamines, see page 49. Do not use this drug without consulting your doctor if your child has heart or thyroid disease or if symptoms are accompanied by high fever or difficulty in breathing. If no improvement in 7 days, consult your doctor. Dosage for children 12 years of age or over: 2 capsules every 6 hours, up to 8 capsules daily; for dosage for children under 12 years of age, consult your doctor. Common side effects: excitability, drowsiness. *Warning:* Should the latter side effect occur, deter your child from engaging in any potentially hazardous activity which requires alertness.

√ *CORICIDIN* (OTC). Tablets. Treats symptoms of common cold and the flu. Chlorpheniramine maleate (antihistamine) and aspirin (analgesic, antipyretic). For profiles of antihistamines and aspirin, see pages 49 and 151, respectively. Do not use without consulting your doctor if your child has asthma, glaucoma, difficulty urinating, stomach distress, ulcers or bleeding problems, or is sensitive to aspirin. Do not use this drug if your child is taking a prescription blood thinner (anticoagulant) or a drug to treat diabetes, gout, or arthritis. Dosage for children 12 years of age or over, 2 tablets every 4 hours, up to 12 tablets in 24 hours; for children 6 to 12 years of age, 1 tablet every 4 hours, up to 5 tablets in 24 hours; for dosages for children under 6 years of age, consult your doctor. Have child drink a full glass of water with each dose. If your child is 6 to 12 years of age, do not give this drug for more than 5 days; and if fever persists for more than 3 days, discontinue use and consult your doctor. Common side effects are excitability, ringing in the ears, drowsiness. If ringing in the ears occurs, discontinue use of this drug and consult your doctor. If drowsiness occurs, deter your child from engaging in any potentially hazardous activity requiring alertness.

√ *CORICIDIN Children's Cough Syrup* (OTC). For relief of cough symptoms and stuffy nose. Dextromethorphan hydrochloride (antitussive), phenylpropanolamine hydrochloride (decongestant), guaifenesin (expectorant), and alcohol (sedative and solvent). Do not use with out consulting your doctor if your child has high blood pressure, heart disease, diabetes, or thyroid disease. Should cough persist or be accompanied by high fever, rash, or a headache that won't go away, discontinue use and consult your doctor. Do not use if your child is taking a prescription antihypertensive (drug to lower blood pressure) or an antidepressant containing a MAO (monoamine oxidase) inhibitor. Dosage

75

for children 6 to 12 years of age, 2 teaspoons every 4 hours, up to 12 teaspoons in 24 hours; for children 2 to 6 years of age, 1 teaspoon every 4 hours, up to 6 teaspoons in 24 hours. The manufacturer reports no side effects at these dosages.

CORICIDIN Cough Syrup (OTC). Fruit-flavored. For coughs commonly associated with colds and flu. Dextromethor-phan hydrobromide (antitussive), phenylpropanolamine hydrochloride (decongestant), guaifenesin (expectorant), alcohol (sedative and solvent). Do not use without consult-ing your doctor if your child has high blood pressure, heart disease, diabetes, or thyroid disease. Do not use this drug if your child is taking a prescription antihypertensive (drug to lower blood pressure) or antidepressant containing a MAO (monoamine oxidase) inhibitor. Dosage for children 12 years of age or over, 2 teaspoons every 4 hours; children 6 to 11 years of age, 1 teaspoons every 4 hours; children 2 to 5 years of age, ½ teaspoon every 4 hours; in no case use more than 6 doses a day. Do not use in children under 2 years of age. The manufacturer reports no side effects at these dosages.

CORICIDIN D (OTC). Decongestant tablets. For congested cold, flu. Chlorpheniramine maleate (antihistamine), phe-nylpropanolamine hydrochloride (decongestant). See CORI-CIDIN in this section. Do not use this drug if your child is taking a prescription blood thinner (anticoagulant); an antihypertensive (drug to lower blood pressure); an anti-depressant containing a MAO (monoamine oxidase) inhib-itor; or a drug to treat diabetes, gout, or arthritis.

CORICIDIN Decongestant Nasal Mist (OTC). For relief of nasal congestion due to common cold. Phenylephrine hydrochloride (decongestant). Dosage for children 12 years of age or over, spray 2 or 3 times in each nostril every 4 hours. Manufacturer reports no side effects at this dosage.

√ *CORICIDIN DEMILETS Tablets for Children* (OTC). For relief of congested cold and flu symptoms. Chlorphenira-mine maleate (antihistamine), aspirin (analgesic and antipy-retic), phenylpropanolamine hydrochloride (deconges-tant). Do not use without consulting your doctor if your child has asthma, glaucoma, difficulty urinating, stomach distress, ulcers or bleeding problems, high blood pressure, heart disease, diabetes, or thyroid disease. Do not use this drug if your child is taking a prescription blood thinner (anticoagulant); a hypertensive (drug to lower blood pres-sure); an antidepressant containing a MAO (monoamine oxidase) inhibitor; or a drug to treat diabetes, gout, or arthritis. Dosage for children 6 to 12 years of age, 2 tablets every 4 hours, up to 12 tablets in 14 hours; for children under 6 years of age, consult your physician. Water must be taken with each dose. Common side effects include excita-bility and drowsiness. *Warning:* Should signs of drowsiness occur, deter your child from engaging in any potentially hazardous activity requiring alertness.

√ *CORICIDIN MEDILETS Tablets for Children* (OTC). For relief of cold and flu symptoms. Chlorpheniramine maleate (antihistamine), aspirin (analgesic, antipyretic). For profiles of antihistamines and aspirin, see pages 49 and 151, respec-tively. Do not use without consulting your doctor if your child has asthma, glaucoma, difficulty urinating, stomach distress (nausea, stomach pain, stomach cramps, belching), ulcers or bleeding problems, or is sensitive to aspirin. Do not use this drug if your child is taking a prescription blood thinner (anticoagulant) or a drug to treat diabetes, gout, or arthritis. Dosage for children 6 to 12 years of age, 2 tablets every 4 hours, up to 12 tablets in 24 hours; for children under 6 years of age, consult your doctor. Give water with each dose. Do not use this drug for more than 3 days if fever persists or occurs, and not for more than 5 days in any case. Common side effects include ringing in the ears and drowsiness. *Warning:* If ringing in the ears occurs, discontinue use and consult your doctor. If drowsiness occurs, deter your child from engaging in any potentially hazardous activity requiring alertness.

√ *FORMULA 44* (OTC). Syrup. For relief of coughs due to colds, flu, and bronchitis. Dextromethorphan hydrobromide (antitussive), doxylamine succinate (antihistamine), sodium citrate (antitussive), and alcohol (sedative and solvent). For a profile of antihistamines, see page 49. Do not use if child has a persistent cough, high fever, or if there is no relief after 3 days. Dosage for children 6 to 12 years of age, 1 teaspoon repeated every 4 hours as needed, up to 6 doses a day. The most common side effect is drowsiness. Should it occur, deter your child from engaging in any potentially hazardous activity requiring alertness. Other possible side effects include nausea, vomiting, dizziness, headache, and clumsiness.

√ *FORMULA 44D Decongestant Cough Mixture* (OTC). Cherry-flavored syrup. For relief of congested cold and flu symptoms. Dextromethorphan hydrobromide (antitussive), phenylpropanolamine hydrochloride (decongestant), guaifenesin (expectorant). Do not use this drug without consulting your doctor if your child has a high fever, persistent cough, high blood pressure, heart disease, diabetes, or thyroid disease. Dosage, no more than 6 doses a day, repeated every 4 hours as needed, for children 6 to 12 years of age, 1 teaspoon; for children 2 to 6 years of age, ½ teaspoon. The manufacturer reports no side effects at these dosages.

HEADWAY CAPSULES/TABLETS (OTC). For colds, sinus, allergy. Acetaminophen (analgesic, antipyretic), phenylpropanolamine hydrochloride (decongestant). Do not use this drug without consulting your physician if your child has high fever, asthma, glaucoma, high blood pressure, heart disease, diabetes, difficulty urinating, or thyroid disease. Do not use for more than 10 days. Dosage, no more than 4 a day, repeated every 4 hours, for children 6 to 12 years of age, 1 capsule or tablet. Do not give to children under 6 years of age without approval of your physician. Side effects: excitability and drowsiness. *Warning:* Should the latter symptom occur, deter your child from engaging in any potentially hazardous activity requiring alertness.

√ *HYCOMINE PEDIATRIC* (℞). Syrup. To treat cough and congestion due to colds and other causes. Hydrocodone bitartrate (analgesic, antitussive), phenylpropanolamine (decongestant). Do not use this drug if your child is sensitive to either ingredient. Your doctor may not prescribe this drug if your child has diabetes, high blood pressure, or thyroid or heart disease. Dosage for children 6 to 12 years of age, 1 teaspoon after meals and at bedtime, not more than every 4 hours, up to 6 teaspoons in 24 hours. Common side effects: heart palpitations, stomach upset, nervousness, dizziness, drowsiness. *Warning:* Should drowsiness occur, deter your child from engaging in any potentially hazardous activity requiring alertness. May be addictive. ☑ Not approved by the FDA.

NALDECON-CX SUSPENSION (OTC). Liquid. For relief of cough and nasal congestion due to colds and other causes. Phenylpropanolamine hydrochloride (decongestant), guaifenesin (expectorant), codeine phosphate (antitussive). For a profile of codeine, see page 72. Do not use if your child is sensitive to any of the ingredients or chemical relatives of phenylpropanolamine hydrochloride (consult your doctor). Do not use without consulting your doctor if your child has high blood pressure, heart disease, diabetes, thyroid disease, asthma, emphysema, or if your child is taking a prescription drug containing a MAO (monoamine oxidase) inhibitor. Should cough persist for 1 week or be accompanied by high fever, rash, or a headache that won't go away, consult your doctor. Dosage: for children over 12 years of age, 2 teaspoons 4 times a day; for children 6 to 12 years of age, 1 teaspoon 4 times a day; for children 2 to 6 years of age, ½ teaspoon 4 times a day. The manufacturer reports no side effects at these dosages.

√ *NALDECON-DX Pediatric Syrup* (OTC). For relief of cough and nasal congestion due to colds and other causes. Dextromethorphan hydrobromide (antitussive), phenylpropanolamine hydrochloride (decongestant), guaifenesin (expectorant), alcohol (sedative and solvent). See NALDECON-CX SUSPENSION in this section. This drug does not contain codeine. Dosage for children over 6 years, 2 teaspoons 4 times daily; for children 2 to 6 years old, 1 teaspoon 4 times daily. The manufacturer reports no side effects at these dosages.

√ *NALDECON-EX Pediatric Drops* (OTC). Decongestant/ex pectorant of special value to infants with colds. Phenylpropanolamine hydrochloride (decongestant), guaifenesin (expectorant), alcohol (sedative and solvent). Do not use without consulting your doctor if your child has high blood pressure, heart disease, diabetes, thyroid disease, asthma, emphysema, or if your child is taking a prescription drug containing a MAO (monoamine oxidase) inhibitor. Should cough persist for 1 week or be accompanied by a high fever, rash, or a headache that won't go away, discontinue use and consult your doctor. Dosage for children, to be given 4 times a day—10 months of age or over (21 lb. or more), 1 ml.; 7 to 9 months of age (18 to 20 lb.), ¾ ml.; 4 to 5 months of age (13 to 17 lb.), ½ ml.; 1 month to 3 months of age (8 to 12 lb.), ¼ ml. For children under 2 years of age, use only as directed by a doctor. This drug comes with a calibrated dropper (a dropper that supplies exact dosages). The manufacturer reports no side effects at recommended dosages.

NALDECON Pediatric Syrup (OTC). See NALDECON Tablets in this section. Dosage for children 3 to 6 months of age, ¼ ml. drops every 3 to 4 hours, up to 4 doses every 24 hours; children 6 to 12 months of age, ½ ml. drops or ½ teaspoon every 3 to 4 hours, up to 4 doses every 24 hours; children 1 year to 6 years of age, 1 ml. drops or 1 teaspoon every 3 to 4 hours, up to 4 doses every 24 hours. ☑ Not approved by the FDA.

NALDECON Syrup (℞). See NALDECON Tablets in this section. Dosage for children 6 to 12 years of age, ½ teaspoon every 3 to 4 hours, up to 4 doses in 24 hours; for children over 12 years of age, 1 teaspoon every 3 to 4 hours, up to 4 doses in 24 hours. ☑ Not approved by the FDA.

NALDECON Tablets (sustained-release) (℞). For the relief of cold symptoms and other disorders. Phenylpropanolamine hydrochloride (decongestant), phenylephrine hydrochloride (decongestant), phenyltoloxamine citrate (antihistamine), chlorpheniramine maleate (antihistamine). For a profile of antihistamines, see page 49. Your doctor will not prescribe this drug if your child is sensitive to any of its ingredients. Your doctor may not prescribe this drug if your child has high blood pressure, glaucoma, diabetes, a type of blood vessel disease, or heart or thyroid disease, or if your child is taking a CNS depressant (see page 225). Dosage for children 6 to 12 years of age, ½ tablet 3 times daily; for children over 12 years of age, 1 tablet 3 times daily. Common side effects: stomach upset, anxiety, drowsiness. *Warning:* If signs of drowsiness occur, deter your child from any potentially hazardous activity requiring alertness. ☑ Not approved by the FDA.

NOVAFED Capsules (℞). Controlled-release decongestant. For continuous 12-hour relief of nasal and eustachian tube (ear) congestion. The eustachian tube is that part of the auditory system which connects the middle ear to the pharynx (the throat). Pseudoephedrine hydrochloride (decongestant). Your doctor will not prescribe this drug if your child is sensitive to this or chemically related drugs (consult your physician), has severe high blood pressure or coronary artery disease, or is taking a MAO (monoamine oxidase) inhibitor. Your doctor may not prescribe this drug if your child has any indication of high blood pressure, diabetes, a certain type of heart disease (deficiency of blood), pressure in the ear, or hyperthyroidism. This drug decreases the blood-pressure-lowering (antihypertensive) effects of certain drugs (consult your physician). Dosage for children over 12 years of age, 1 capsule every 12 hours. Common side effects: nausea, vomiting, sleeping, breathing or urinating difficulties, tenseness, nervousness, trembling, restlessness, headaches, dizziness.

NOVAFED-A Capsules (℞). Controlled-release decongestant plus antihistamine. Provides about 12 hours' relief from nasal and eustachian tube congestion from colds and other causes. (See NOVAFED Capsules.) Pseudoephedrine hydrochloride (decongestant), chlorpheniramine maleate (antihistamine). For a profile of antihistamines, see page 49. Your doctor will not prescribe this drug if your child has asthma, is sensitive to the drug's ingredients, has severe high blood pressure, severe coronary heart disease, narrow-angle glaucoma, peptic ulcer, or urinary retention, or is taking a MAO (monoamine oxidase) inhibitor. Dosage for children over 12 years of age, 1 capsule every 12 hours. Common side effects: nausea; vomiting; sleeping, breathing or urinating difficulties; tenseness; nervousness; trembling; restlessness; headaches; dizziness; blurred vision; drowsiness. *Warning:* Should signs of drowsiness occur, deter your child from engaging in any potentially hazardous activity requiring alertness. ☑ Not approved by the FDA.

NOVAFED-A Decongestant Plus Antihistamine Liquid (OTC). See NOVAFED-A Capsules; add alcohol (sedative and solvent) to list of ingredients. Dosage for children over 12 years of age, 2 teaspoons every 4 hours; for children 6 to 12 years of age, 1 teaspoon every 4 hours; for children under 6 years of age, consult your physician. Maximum of 4 doses in 24 hours.

NOVAFED Liquid (OTC). See NOVAFED Capsules in this section. Dosage for children over 12 years of age, 2 teaspoons every 4 hours; children 6 to 12 years of age, 1 teaspoon every 4 hours; children 2 to 5 years of age, ½ teaspoon every 4 hours; 4 doses in 24 hours is maximum permitted in these age groups. For dosage for children under 2 years of age, consult your doctor.

NOVAHISTINE COLD TABLETS (OTC). For relief of cold symptoms, except cough and fever. Phenylpropanolamine hydrochloride (decongestant), chlorpheniramine maleate (antihistamine). For a profile of antihistamines, see page 49. Do not use if your child has severe high blood pressure, coronary disease, narrow-angle glaucoma, urinary retention, peptic ulcer, or asthma. Your doctor may not approve use of this drug if your child has any degree of high blood pressure, a certain disease of the heart (deficiency of blood), increased pressure inside the ears, diabetes, or hyperthyroidism. Effects of this drug are increased by

MAO (monoamine oxidase) inhibitors (therefore, do not use this drug if child is taking such an inhibitor); effects of certain drugs to lower blood pressure are decreased by this drug. Dosages for children 6 to 12 years of age, 1 tablet every 4 hours, no more than 4 doses in 24 hours; for children under 6 years of age, consult your doctor.

NOVAHISTINE COUGH FORMULA Antitussive-Expectorant Liquid (OTC). For dry coughs associated with colds, flu, and pertussis (whooping cough). Dextromethorphan hydrobromide (antitussive), guaifenesin (expectorant). Do not use if child is sensitive to any ingredient of this drug, has a chronic cough, asthma, or other serious respiratory disorder, or is taking a MAO (monoamine oxidase) inhibitor or any of the following drugs: penicillins; tetracyclines; salicylates; phenobarbital; or iodides in high concentrations. Dosage for children 12 years of age or older, 2 teaspoons every 4 hours; for children 6 to 12 years of age, 1 teaspoon every 4 hours; for children 2 to under 6 years of age, ½ teaspoon every 2 hours; for children under 2 years of age, consult your doctor; maximum: 4 doses in 24 hours.

NOVAHISTINE COUGH & COLD FORMULA Antitussive-Decongestant Liquid (OTC). Dextromethorphan hydrobromide (antitussive), pseudoephedrine hydrochloride (decongestant), chlorpheniramine maleate (antihistamine), alcohol (sedative and solvent). For a profile of antihistamines, see page 49. Do not use if child has a chronic cough, has asthma (never use during an asthmatic attack) or other serious respiratory disorder, narrow-angle glaucoma, urinary retention, peptic ulcer, severe high blood pressure, or coronary heart disease. Your doctor may not approve use of this drug if your child is diabetic, has any degree of high blood pressure, is hyperactive to ephedrine, or has any cardiovascular disease. Effects of this drug are increased by MAO (monoamine oxidase) inhibitors and beta blockers (beta andrenergic blockers); effects of certain drugs to lower blood pressure are decreased by this drug. Dosage for children 12 years of age or older, 2 teaspoons every 4 to 6 hours; children 6 to under 12 years of age, 1 teaspoon every 4 to 6 hours; for children under 6 years of age, consult your physician; not more than 4 doses in 24 hours. Common side effects: nausea, vomiting, stomach upset, drowsiness. *Warning:* Should signs of drowsiness occur, deter your child from any potentially hazardous activity which requires alertness.

NOVAHISTINE DH Liquid (OTC). For relief of coughs and nasal congestion due to colds and other causes. Codeine phosphate (antitussive), phenylpropanolamine hydrochloride (decongestant), chlorpheniramine maleate (antihistamine). For profiles of codeine and antihistamines, see pages 79 and 49, respectively. Do not use if your child has severe high blood pressure or coronary heart disease, narrow-angle glaucoma, urinary retention, peptic ulcer, asthma, or is sensitive to any of the drug's ingredients. Your doctor may not prescribe this drug if your child has any degree of high blood pressure, diabetes, a certain type of heart disease (deficiency of blood), increased pressure inside the ear, hyperthyroidism, other thyroid disorders, or emphysema. Effects of this drug are increased by MAO (monoamine oxidase) inhibitors (therefore, do not use if your child is taking any of these inhibitors) and by beta blockers (beta andrenergic blockers); effects of certain drugs to lower blood pressure are decreased by this drug. Dosage for children 6 to 12 years of age, 1 teaspoon every 4 hours; for children 2 to 5 years of age, ½ teaspoon every 4 hours; do not exceed 4 doses in 24 hours. Common side effects: nausea, vomiting, constipation, dizziness, palpitations, tenseness, restlessness, anxiety, difficulties urinating. May be addictive. ☑ Not approved by the FDA.

NOVAHISTINE DMX Antitussive-Decongestant Liquid (OTC). Dextromethorphan hydrobromide (antitussive), pseudoephedrine hydrochloride (decongestant), guaifenesin (expectorant). For a dry cough associated with colds, flu, bronchitis, and sinusitis. Do not use if your child is sensitive to any ingredient of the drug or has severe coronary heart disease or high blood pressure. Your doctor may not approve use of this drug if your child has any degree of high blood pressure, a certain type of heart disease (deficiency of blood), pressure inside the ears, diabetes, or hyperthyroidism. Effects of this drug are increased by MAO (monoamine oxidase) inhibitors and beta blockers (beta andrenergic blockers); effects of certain drugs to lower blood pressure are decreased by this drug. Dosages for children 6 to 12 years of age, 1 teaspoon every 4 to 6 hours; for children 2 to 5 years of age, ½ teaspoon every 4 to 6 hours; for children under 2 years of age, consult your doctor; not more than 4 doses in 24 hours. Common side effects: nausea, stomach upset.

√ *NOVAHISTINE ELIXIR* (OTC). See NOVAHISTINE COLD TABLETS in this section. Dosages for children 6 to 12 years of age, 1 teaspoon every 4 hours; no more than 4 doses in 24 hours; for children under 12 years of age, consult your doctor.

NOVAHISTINE EXPECTORANT (OTC). Liquid. For loosening hard-to-loosen secretions of the lungs associated with cough. Codeine phosphate (antitussive), phenylpropanolamine hydrochloride (decongestant), guaifenesin (expectorant), alcohol (sedative and solvent). See NOVAHISTINE DH Liquid in this section. Novahistine Expectorant, though, does not contain an antihistamine. Dosage for children 50 to 90 pounds, ½ to 1 teaspoon every 4 hours; children 25 to 50 pounds, ¼ to ½ teaspoon every 4 hours; children under 2 years of age, 3 drops per kilogram (about 2.2 lb.) every 4 hours; no more than 4 doses in 24 hours. ☑ Not approved by the FDA.

NYQUIL Nightime Cold Medicine (OTC). Anise-flavored syrup. Helps permit sleep by relieving symptoms of a cold. Acetaminophen (analgesic and antipyretic), doxylamine succinate (antihistamine), ephedrine sulfate (decongestant), dextromethorphan hydrobromide (antitussive), alcohol (sedative and solvent), FD 8C Yellow No. 5 (tartrazine, a coloring agent). The alcohol content (2.5 percent) is higher than in most colds medicines. For a profile of antihistamines, see page 49. Do not use without approval of your doctor if your child has high blood pressure, heart disease, diabetes, thyroid disease, high fever, or persistent cough. Dosage for children 10 to 12 years of age, 1 tablespoon at bedtime; except if confined or at home, 1 dose every 4 hours is permitted, but not more than 4 doses in 24 hours. Common side effects: nervousness, restlessness, sleeplessness.

√ *ORNADE 2 LIQUID FOR CHILDREN* (OTC). To relieve symptoms of nasal congestion. Phenylpropanolamine hydrochloride (decongestant), chlorpheniramine maleate (antihistamine), alcohol (sedative and solvent). For a profile of antihistamines, see page 49. Do not use if your child is sensitive to ingredients of this drug, has severe high blood pressure, coronary heart disease, asthma, or is taking a MAO (monoamine oxidase) inhibitor or a prescription antihypertensive (a drug to lower blood pressure). Your doctor may not approve use of this drug if your child has any degree of high blood pressure, heart disease, diabetes, or thyroid disease. Dosage for children 12 years of age or over, 2 teaspoons every 4 hours; for children 6 to 12 years of age, 1 teaspoon every 4 hours; for children 2 to 6 years of age, ½ teaspoon every 4 to 6 hours; do not exceed 6 doses in 24 hours. Common side effects are nervousness, sleeplessness, dizziness, drowsiness. *Warning:* If signs of drowsiness occur, deter your child from engaging in any potentially hazardous activity requiring alertness.

PEDIACOF Decongestant and Soothing Cough Syrup for Children (℞). For the relief of coughs and congestion due to colds and other causes. Codeine phosphate (antitussive), phenylephrine hydrochloride (decongestant), chlorpheniramine maleate (antihistamine), potassium iodide (antitussive), alcohol (solvent and sedative), and sodium benzoate (preservative). For profiles of codeine and antihistamines, see pages 79 and 49, respectively. Do not use if your child is sensitive to any of the ingredients of this drug or has tuberculosis, ventricular tachycardia (a heart disorder), or severe hypertension. Your doctor may not prescribe this drug if your child has any type of heart disorder, any degree of high blood pressure, or hyperthyroidism. This drug acts on CNS depressants much as barbiturates (see page 35). Dosages for children 6 to 12 years of age, 2 teaspoons every 4 to 6 hours; for children 3 to 6 years of age, 1 teaspoon to 2 teaspoons every 4 to 6 hours; for children 1 year to 3 years of age, ½ to 1 teaspoon every 4 to 6 hours; for children 6 months to 1 year of age, ¼ teaspoon every 4 to 6 hours. Common side effects: loss of appetite, constipation, drowsiness. *Warning:* Should signs of drowsiness occur, deter your child from engaging in any activity requiring alertness. ☑ Not approved by the FDA.

/ *PHENERGAN EXPECTORANT WITH DEXTROMETHORPHAN PEDIATRIC* (℞). Syrup. For the relief of coughs due to colds and other causes. Dextromethorphan hydrobromide (antitussive), promethazine hydrochloride (antihistamine), fluid extract ipecac (expectorant), potassium guaiacolsulfonate (expectorant), citric acid (expectorant), and sodium citrate(expectorant). Do not use if your child is sensitive to guaifenesin. Acts like barbiturates on CNS depressants, including barbiturates (see page 35). Dosage for children over 4 years, 1 teaspoon to 2 teaspoons in 1 dose to 4 doses a day, no less than 3 hours apart; for children 3 months to 4 years, ½ teaspoon in 1 dose to 4 doses a day, no less than 3 hours apart. Common side effects: dry mouth, blurred vision, dizziness, drowsiness. *Warning:* Should signs of drowsiness occur, deter your child from engaging in any potentially hazardous activity requiring alertness.

ROBITUSSIN (OTC). Syrup. For the relief of cough due to the common cold and other causes. Guaifenesin (expectorant), alcohol (sedative and solvent). Do not use if your child is sensitive to guaifenesin. Dosage for children 12 years of age or over, 2 teaspoons every 4 hours, not to exceed 12 teaspoons in 24 hours; for children 6 to 11 years of age, 1 teaspoon every 4 hours, not to exceed 6 teaspoons in 24 hours; for children 2 to 6 years of age, ½ teaspoon every 4 hours, not to exceed 3 teaspoons in 24 hours; for children under 2 years of age, consult your physician. The manufacturer reports no serious side effects.

ROBITUSSIN A-C (OTC). Syrup. For the relief of cough due to the common cold and other causes. Guaifenesin (expectorant), codeine phosphate (antitussive), alcohol (sedative and solvent). For a profile of codeine, see page 79. Do not use if child is sensitive to any of the ingredients of this drug. Do not use without your doctor's approval if your child has a persistent or chronic cough, certain respiratory diseases, or shortness of breath. Acts like barbiturates on CNS depressants, including barbiturates (see page 35). Dosage for children 12 years of age or over, 2 teaspoons every 4 hours, up to 6 teaspoons in 24 hours; for children 2 to 6 years of age, ½ teaspoon every 4 hours, up to 3 teaspoons in 24 hours; for children under 2 years of age, consult your doctor. Common side effects: constipation, upset stomach, nausea, drowsiness. *Warning:* Should signs of drowsiness occur, deter your child from engaging in any potentially hazardous activity requiring alertness. May be addictive.

√ *ROBITUSSIN-CF* (OTC). Syrup. For the relief of cough due to the common cold and other causes. Guaifenesin (expectorant), phenylpropanolamine hydrochloride (decongestant), dextromethorphan hydrobromide (antitussive), alcohol (sedative and solvent). Do not use if your child is sensitive to any ingredient of this drug, has severe high blood pressure or hyperthyroidism, or is receiving MAO (monoamine oxidase) inhibitors or anti-high-blood-pressure medicine. Dosage is the same as for Robitussin. Common side effects: nausea, vomiting, dry mouth, nervousness, sleeplessness, restlessness, headache.

ROBITUSSIN-DAC (OTC). Syrup. For the relief of cough and nasal congestion due to colds or inhaled irritants. Guaifenesin hydrochloride (decongestant), pseudoephedrine hydrochloride (decongestant), codeine phosphate (antitussive). For a profile of codeine, see page 79. Do not use if your child is sensitive to any ingredient of this drug, has hyperthyroidism, severe hypertension, or is receiving MAO (monoamine oxidase) inhibitors or anti-high-blood-pressure medicine. Dosages for children 12 years of age or over, 1 teaspoon to 2 teaspoons every 4 hours, not to exceed 4 teaspoons in 24 hours; for children 2 to 6 years of age, ½ teaspoon every 4 hours, not to exceed 2 teaspoons in 24 hours; for children under 2 years, consult your doctor. Common side effects: constipation, nausea, sleeplessness, restlessness, palpitations. May be addictive.

ROBITUSSIN-DM (OTC). Syrup. For the relief of cough due to the common cold and other causes. Guaifenesin (expectorant), dextromethorphan hydrobromide (antitussive), alcohol (sedative and solvent). Do not use if your child is sensitive to any ingredient of this drug or is receiving MAO (monoamine oxidase) inhibitors. Dosage for children 12 years of age or over, 2 teaspoons every 6 to 8 hours, not to exceed 8 teaspoons in 24 hours; for children 6 to 12 years of age, 1 teaspoon every 6 to 8 hours, not to exceed 4 teaspoons in 24 hours; for children 2 to 6 years of age, ½ teaspoon every 6 to 8 hours, not to exceed 2 teaspoons in 24 hours; for children under 2 years of age, consult your doctor. The manufacturer reports no serious side effects.

ROBITUSSIN-PE (OTC). For the relief of cough due to the common cold and other causes. Guaifenesin (expectorant), pseudoephedrine hydrochloride (decongestant). See RO-BITUSSIN-CF in this section for "do not use" instructions. Dosage for children 12 years of age or over, 2 teaspoons every 4 hours, not to exceed 8 teaspoons in 24 hours; for children 6 to 12 years of age, 1 teaspoon every 4 hours, not to exceed 4 teaspoon in 24 hours; for children 2 to 6 years of age, ½ teaspoon every 4 hours, not to exceed 2 teaspoons in 24 hours; for children under 2 years of age, consult your doctor. For common side effects, see RO-BITUSSIN-CF.

√ *RONDEC* Drops for Infants. For relief of symptoms of the common cold, including postnasal drip, and symptoms of other respiratory diseases. Carbinoxamine maleate (antihistamine), pseudoephedrine hydrochloride (decongestant). For a profile of antihistamines, see page 49. Your doctor may not prescribe this drug if your child is sensitive to any of its ingredients, has high blood pressure, asthma, diabetes, heart or thyroid disease, or is receiving CNS depressants or

MAO (monoamine oxidase) inhibitors. Dosage for infants 9 to 18 months, 1 dropperful 4 times a day; for infants 6 to 9 months, ¾ dropperful 4 times a day; for infants 3 to 6 months, ½ dropperful 4 times a day; for infants 1 month to 3 months, ¼ dropperful 4 times a day. Common side effects: stimulation or drowsiness. *Warning:* If signs of drowsiness occur, deter your child from engaging in any potentially hazardous activity requiring alertness. ☑ Not approved by the FDA.

RONDEC Syrup for Young Children (℞). See RONDEC Drops for Infants in this section. Dosage for children 6 years of age or older, 1 teaspoon 4 times a day; for children 18 months of age to 6 years, ½ teaspoon 4 times a day. ☑Not approved by the FDA.

RONDEC Tablets (℞). For adults and for children 6 years or over. See RONDEC Drops for Infants in this section. Dosage for children 6 years of age or over, 1 tablet 4 times a day. ☑Not approved by the FDA.

√ *RONDEC-DM™ Drops* (℞). See RONDEC-DM™ Syrup. Dosage for children 9 to 18 months of age, 1 dropperful 4 times a day; for children 6 to 9 months of age, ¾ dropperful 4 times a day; for children 3 to 6 months, ½ dropperful 4 times a day; for children 1 month to 3 months, ¼ dropperful 4 times a day. ☑Not approved by the FDA.

√ *RONDEC-DM™ Syrup* (℞). For the relief of symptoms of the common cold, postnasal drip, and similar maladies. Carbinoxamine maleate (histamine), pseudoephedrine hydrochloride (decongestant), dextromethorphan hydrobromide (antitussive), alcohol (sedative and solvent). For a profile of antihistamines, see page 49. Do not use if your child is sensitive to any ingredient of this drug or has narrow-angle glaucoma, urinary retention, peptic ulcer, severe high blood pressure, coronary heart disease, asthma, or is receiving MAO (monoamine oxidase) inhibitors or beta blockers (beta andrenergic blockers). Your doctor may not prescribe this drug if your child has any degree of high blood pressure, heart disease, asthma, hyperthyroidism, increased pressure in the inner ear, or diabetes. This drug acts like barbiturates on CNS depressants, including barbiturates (see page 35). Dosage for children 6 years of age or over, 1 teaspoon 4 times a day; for children 18 months to 6 years of age, ½ teaspoon 4 times a day. Common side effects: mild gastrointestinal disturbances, stimulation, drowsiness. *Warning:* If signs of drowsiness occur, deter your child from engaging in potentially hazardous activities requiring alertness. ☑ Not approved by the FDA.

RONDEC-TR Tablets (℞). For adults and children 12 years of age or over. See RONDEC Drops for Infants in this section. Dosage for children 12 years of age or over, 1 tablet 2 times a day. ☑ Not approved by the FDA.

RYNATUSS Pediatric Suspension (℞). For relief of cough associated with the common cold and similar maladies. Carbetapentane tannate (antitussive), chlorpheniramine tannate (antihistamine), ephidrene tannate (decongestant), FD 8C Yellow No. 5 (tartrazine, a coloring agent). For a profile of antihistamines, see page 49. Do not use this drug if your child is sensitive to any of its ingredients. Your doctor may not prescribe this drug if your child is sensitive to any of its ingredients. Your doctor may not prescribe this drug if your child has high blood pressure, cardiovascular disease, hyperthyroidism, narrow-angle glaucoma, diabetes, or is receiving MAO (monoamine oxidase) inhibitors. This drug acts like barbiturates on CNS depressants, including barbiturates (see page 35). FD 8C Yellow No. 5 can cause allergic reactions, including bronchial asthma, particularly if your child is sensitive to aspirin. Dosage for children over 6 years of age, 1 teaspoon to 2 teaspoons; for children under 2 years of age, consult your doctor. Common side effects: dry mouth, drowsiness. *Warning:* Should signs of drowsiness occur, deter your child from engaging in potentially hazardous activities requiring alertness. ☑ Not approved by the FDA.

√ *ST. JOSEPH ASPIRIN FOR CHILDREN* (OTC). Orange-flavored chewable tablets. For the relief of headache and painful discomfort of the common cold, and for other uses. For a profile of aspirin (analgesic, antipyretic), see page 151. Manufacturer does not report any adverse side effects at recommended dosages.

√ *ST. JOSEPH COLD TABLETS FOR CHILDREN* (OTC). Orange-flavored. For relief of minor aches and pains, fever, and nasal congestion due to colds. Aspirin (analgesic, antipyretic), and phenylpropanolamine hydrochloride (decongestant). For a profile on aspirin, see page 151. Consult your doctor under the following conditions: if symptoms persist for more than 5 days (under any circumstance, discontinue use of this drug after 5 days); if fever persists for more than 3 days; if sore throat accompanied by high fever, headaches, nausea, or vomiting persists for 24 hours. Manufacturer does not report any adverse side effects at recommended dosages.

√ *ST. JOSEPH COUGH SYRUP FOR CHILDREN* (OTC). Cherry-flavored. For the relief of cough of colds and flu for up to 8 hours. Dextromethorphan hydrobromide (antitussive). Do not use without your doctor's approval if your child has a persistent or chronic cough associated with asthma or emphysema, or if cough is accompanied by excess secretions. Dosage for children 12 years of age or older (84 lb. or more of body weight), 4 teaspoons every 6 to 8 hours, up to 16 teaspoons daily; for children 6 to under 12 years of age (46 to 83 lb. of body weight), 2 teaspoons every 6 to 8 hours, up to 8 teaspoons daily; for children 2 to under 6 years (27 to 45 lb. of body weight), 1 teaspoon every 6 to 8 hours, up to 4 teaspoons daily; for children under 2 years of age (below 27 lb. of body weight), consult your doctor. The manufacturer reports no adverse side effects at these dosages.

SINUBID (R). Tablets. For the relief of symptoms of the common cold and other disorders. Acetaminophen (analgesic, antipyretic), phenacetin (analgesic, antipyretic), phenylpropanolamine hydrochloride (decongestant), phenyltoloxamine citrate (antihistamine). For a profile of antihistamines, see page 49. Do not use if your child is sensitive to any ingredient of this drug. Your doctor may not prescribe this drug if your child has high blood pressure, chronic kidney disease, diabetes, or heart or thyroid disease. Acts like barbiturates on CNS depressants, including barbiturates (see page 35) and increases the effects of MAO (monoamine oxidase) inhibitors. Dosage for children 6 to 12 years of age, ½ tablet every 12 hours. Common side effects include dry mouth, nausea, vomiting, restlessness, sleeplessness, nervousness, dizziness, clumsiness, and drowsiness. *Warning:* Should signs of drowsiness occur, deter your child from engaging in any potentially hazardous activity requiring alertness.

√ *SUDAFED Cough Syrup* (OTC). For relief of cough and nasal congestion due to colds and flu. Pseudoephedrine hydrochloride (decongestant), dextromethorphan hydrobromide (antitussive), guaifenesin (expectorant). Do not use without your doctor's approval if your child has a persistent or chronic cough associated with asthma or emphysema, if cough is accompanied by excess secretions, or if your child has asthma, glaucoma, high blood pressure, difficulty urinating, diabetes, or heart or thyroid disease. Do not use this drug if your child is taking a prescription anti-high-blood-pressure drug or a MAO (monoamine oxidase) inhibitor. If cough persists for more than 7 days or is accompanied by high fever, rash, or a headache that won't go away, discontinue use and consult your doctor. Dosage for children over 12 years of age, 2 teaspoons every 4 hours; for children 6 to 12 years of age, 1 teaspoon every 4 hours; for children 2 to 5 years of age, ½ teaspoon every 4 hours; for children under 2 years of age, consult your doctor; do not exceed 4 doses in 24 hours. Manufacturer reports no adverse side effects at these dosages; at higher doses, dizziness, nervousness, or sleeplessness may occur.

SUDAFED PLUS SYRUP (OTC). See SUDAFED PLUS TABLETS in this section. Dosage for children over 12 years of age, 2 teaspoons every 4 hours; for children 6 to 12 years of age, 1 teaspoon every 4 hours; do not exceed 4 doses in 24 hours; for children under 6 years of age, consult your doctor.

SUDAFED PLUS TABLETS (OTC). For the relief of the congestion; sneezing; runny nose; and watery, itchy eyes of a common cold. Pseudoephedrine hydrochloride (decongestant) and chlorpheniramine maleate (antihistamine). For a profile of antihistamines, see page 49. Do not use this drug without approval of your doctor if your child has high blood pressure, glaucoma, urinating difficulty, asthma, heart or thyroid disease, or is receiving prescription high-blood-pressure medicine or MAO (monoamine oxidase) inhibitors. If symptoms do not improve within 7 days, discontinue use of this drug and consult your doctor. Dosage for children over 12 years of age, 1 tablet every 4 hours; for children 6 to 12 years of age, ½ tablet every 4 hours; for children under 6 years of age, consult your doctor. Common side effects: excitability and drowsiness. *Warning:* If the latter side effect occurs, deter your child from any potentially hazardous activity requiring alertness.

SUDAFED S.A. CAPSULES (OTC). Sustained-action capsules for relief of congestive cold symptoms for up to 12 hours. See SUDAFED TABLETS in this section. Dosage for children 12 years of age or over, 1 30-mg. capsule every 12 hours.

√ *SUDAFED SYRUP* (OTC). Rasberry-flavored. See SUDAFED TABLETS in this section. Dosage for children 2 to 5 years of age, ½ teaspoon every 4 hours, not to exceed 4 doses in 24 hours; for children under 2 years of age, consult your doctor.

√ *SUDAFED TABLETS,* 30 mg. Sugar-Coated (OTC). For the relief of nasal/sinus congestion. Pseudoephedrine hydrochloride (decongestant). Do not use without the approval of your physician if your child has high blood pressure, urinary retention, glaucoma, or heart or thyroid disease. If symptoms persist for 5 days or are accompanied by high fever, discontinue use of this drug and consult your doctor. Dosage for children over 12 years of age, 2 tablets every 4 hours; for children 6 to 12 years of age, 1 tablet every 4 hours; do not exceed 4 doses in 24 hours. Should common side effects—nausea, headache, sleeplessness, dizziness, nervousness—occur, reduce dosage.

SUDAFED TABLETS, 60 mg. Sugar-Coated Adult Strength (OTC) . See SUDAFED TABLETS 30 mg. Sugar-Coated in this section. Dosage for children over 12 years of age, 1 tablet every 4 hours; do not exceed 4 doses in 24 hours.

TRIAMINIC EXPECTORANT (OTC). Liquid. For relief of cough and nasal congestion due to the common cold. Phenylpropanolamine hydrochloride (decongestant), guaifenesin (expectorant). Do not use without your doctor's approval if your child is sensitive to any ingredient of this drug; has a persistent or chronic cough from chronic asthma, bronchitis, or emphysema; has high blood pressure, heart disease, diabetes, or hyperthyroidism; or is receiving MAO (monoamine oxidase) inhibitors. Dosage for children 6 to 12 years of age, 1 teaspoon every 4 hours; for children 2 to 6 years of age, ½ teaspoon every 4 hours; for children 3 months to 2 years of age, 4 to 5 drops per kilogram (about 2.2 lb.) of weight every 4 hours. Common side effects: stomach upset, nervousness, sleeplessness, dizziness, blurred vision, flushing, palpitations.

TRIAMINIC EXPECTORANT WITH CODEINE (OTC). Liquid. See TRIAMINIC EXPECTORANT, above. For a profile of codeine, see page 79. Dosage for children 6 to 12 years of age, 1 teaspoon every 4 hours; for children 2 to 6 years of age, ¼ teaspoon every 4 hours; for children 3 months to 2 years of age, 2 drops per kilogram (about 2.2 lb.) of body weight every 4 hours. An additional common side effect is constipation. May be addictive.

TRIAMINIC JUVELETS, Timed-Release Tablets (OTC). For relief of nasal congestion and postnasal drip associated with the common cold and other maladies. Phenylpropanolamine hydrochloride (decongestant), pheniramine maleate (antitussive), pyrilamine maleate (antihistamine). For a profile of antihistamines, see page 49. Do not use this drug if your child has severe high blood pressure or coronary heart disease or is receiving MAO (monoamine oxidase) inhibitors, CNS depressants, or certain medicines to lower blood pressure. Your doctor may not prescribe this drug if your child has any degree of high blood pressure, diabetes, cardiovascular disease, narrow-angle glaucoma, a certain type of peptic ulcer, or bladder-neck obstruction. Dosage for children 6 to 12 years of age, 1 tablet 3 times a day (morning, afternoon, bedtime). Common side effects: stomach upset, restlessness, nervousness, drowsiness. *Warning:* If signs of drowsiness occur, deter your child from engaging in any potentially hazardous activity requiring alertness.☑ Not approved by the FDA.

TRIAMINIC ORAL INFANT DROPS (OTC). See TRIAMINIC JUVELETS in this section. Dosage for infants: 1 drop per 2 pounds of body weight 4 times a day. ☑ Not approved by the FDA.

TRIAMINIC SYRUP (OTC). Orange-flavored. To relieve congestion; sneezing; and itchy, watery eyes due to the common cold and other respiratory maladies. Phenylpropanolamine hydrochloride (decongestant), chlorpheniramine hydrochloride (antihistamine). For a profile of antihistamines, see page 49. For a profile of this drug, see TRIAMINIC JUVELETS in this section. Dosage for children 6 to 12 years of age, 1 teaspoon every 4 hours; for children 2 to 6 years of age, ½ teaspoon every 4 hours; for children 3 months to 2 years of age, 4 to 5 drops per kilogram (about 2.2 lb.) of body weight every 4 hours.

TRIAMINIC TABLETS, Timed-Release (OTC). See TRIAMINIC JUVELETS in this section. Dosage for children over 12 years of age, 1 tablet 3 times a day (morning, midafternoon, and bedtime). ☑ Not approved by the FDA.

TRIAMINIC-DM COUGH FORMULA (OTC). For relief of cough and nasal congestion due to the common cold. Phenylpropanolamine hydrochloride (decongestant), dextromethmorphan hydrobromide (antitussive). Do not use this drug if your child is sensitive to any of its ingredients or is receiving MAO (monoamine oxidase) inhibitors. Do not use this drug without your doctor's approval if your child has a persistent or chronic cough associated with bronchitis, asthma, or emphysema, or has heart disease, diabetes, high blood pressure, or hyperthyroidism. Dosage for children 6 to 12 years of age, 1 teaspoon every 4 hours; for children 2 to 6 years of age, ½ teaspoon every 4 hours; for children 3 months to 2 years of age, 1½ drops per kilogram (about 2.2 lb.) of body weight every 4 hours. Common side effects: flushing, stomach upset, palpitations, blurred vision, nervousness, dizziness, sleeplessness.

TRIAMINIC-12™ Sustained-Release Tablets (OTC). For up to 12 hours' relief of congestant symptoms of the common cold and other causes. Phenylpropanolamine hydrochloride (decongestant), chlorpheniramine maleate (antihistamine). For a profile of this drug, see TRIAMINIC JUVELETS in this section. Dosage for children over 12 years of age, 1 tablet every 12 hours; maximum of 2 tablets in 24 hours.

TRIAMINICIN CHEWABLES (OTC). For relief of children's nasal congestion due to the common cold and nasal allergies. Phenylpropanolamine hydrochloride (decongestant), chlorpheniramine maleate (antihistamine). For a profile of antihistamines, see page 49; for a profile of this drug, see TRIAMINIC JUVELETS in this section. Dosage for children 2 to 6 years of age, 1 tablet 4 times a day; for children 6 to 12 years of age, 2 tablets 4 times a day.

TRIAMINICOL DECONGESTANT COUGH SYRUP (OTC). For relief of coughs, especially when accompanied by nasal congestion of the common cold. Phenylpropanolamine (decongestant), chlorpheniramine maleate (antihistamine), pyrilamine maleate (antihistamine), dextromethorphan hydrobromide (antitussive), ammonium chloride (expectorant). For a profile of antihistamines, see page 49. For a profile of this drug, see TRIAMINIC JUVELETS in this section. Dosage for children 6 to 12 years of age, 1 teaspoon every 4 hours; for children 2 to 6 years of age, ½ teaspoon every 4 to 6 hours. ☑ Not approved by the FDA.

TUSSAGESIC SUSPENSION (OTC). For relief of the symptoms of the common cold. Phenylpropanalamine hydrochloride (decongestant), chlorpheniramine maleate (antihistamine), pyrilamine maleate (antihistamine), dextromethorphan hydrobromide (antitussive), terpin hydrate (antitussive), acetominophen (analgesic, antipyretic). For a profile of antihistamines, see page 49. Do not use this drug without approval of your doctor if your child has high blood pressure, heart trouble, diabetes, or hyperthyroidism. Dosage for children 6 to 12 years of age, 1 teaspoon every 4 hours; for children 1 year to 6 years of age, ½ teaspoon every 4 hours.

TUSSEND Antitussive-Decongestant Liquid (℞). For exhausting cough spasms due to the common cold and other respiratory disorders. Hydrocone bitartrate (antitussive), pseudoephedrine hydrochloride (decongestant), alcohol (sedative and solvent). Hydrocone is related chemically to codeine (see page 79). Do not use this drug if your child has a severe respiratory disorder, high blood pressure, diabetes, a type of heart disease (lack of blood), hyperthyroidism, or increased pressure in the inner ear. Do not use this drug if your child is receiving other narcotics, general anesthetics, tranquilizers, sedatives or hypnotics, MAO (monoamine oxidase) inhibitors, alcohol, other CNS depressants, or certain anti-high-blood-pressure drugs. Dosage, given up to 4 times a day as needed, for children over 90 pounds, 1 teaspoon; for children 50 to 90 pounds, ½ teaspoon; for children 25 to 50 pounds, ¼ teaspoon. Common side effects: constipation; stomach upset; nausea; palpitations and other adverse cardiac reactions; difficulty in breathing and urinating; headache; restlessness; nervousness; dizziness; drowsiness. *Warning:* Should signs of drowsiness occur, deter your child from engaging in potentially dangerous activities requiring alertness. May be addictive. ☑ Not approved by the FDA.

TUSSEND Antitussive-Decongestant Tablets (℞). See TUS-SEND Antitussive-Decongestant Liquid in this section. Tablets contain no alcohol. Dosage: Substitute "tablet" for "teaspoon" in Tussend Antitussive Decongestant Liquid entry.

TUSSEND EXPECTORANT (℞). For exhaustive nonproductive cough accompanying the common cold and other respiratory disorders. Hydrocodone bitartrate (antitussive), pseudoephedrine hydrochloride (decongestant), guaifenesin (expectorant). For a profile of this drug, see TUSSEND Antitussive-Decongestant Liquid in this section. ☑ Not approved by the FDA.

TUSSIONEX (OTC). Suspension. For 12-hour relief of nonproductive cough. (A nonproductive cough is one which does not act to clear respiratory passages—a dry cough.) Hydrocodone (antitussive), phenyltoloxamine (antihistamine). Hydrocodone is related chemically to codeine (see page 79). For a profile of antihistamines, see page 49. Your doctor may not prescribe this drug if your child is sensitive to either ingredient, has a severe respiratory disease, or is receiving a CNS depressant. Dosage for children over 5 years of age, 1 teaspoon every 12 hours; for children 1 year to 5 years of age, ½ teaspoon every 12 hours; for children under 1 year of age, ¼ teaspoon every 12 hours.

Common side effects: mild constipation, nausea, facial itching, drowsiness. *Warning:* Should signs of drowsiness occur, deter your child from engaging in potentially dangerous activities requiring alertness. ☑ Not approved by the FDA.

TUSSI-ORGANIDIN™ (℞). Elixir. For the relief of nonproductive cough (see TUSSIONEX in this section) associated with the common cold and other respiratory disorders. Iodinated glycerol (expectorant), codeine phosphate (antitussive), chlorpheniramine maleate (antihistamine), alcohol (sedative and solvent). For profiles of antihistamines and codeine, see pages 49 and 79, respectively. Do not use if your child is sensitive to any ingredient of this drug, or is receiving a CNS depressant, a MAO (monoamine oxidase) inhibitor, lithium, or other antithyroid drugs. Dosage for children, ½ to 1 teaspoon every 4 hours. Common side effects: stomach upset, rash, dry mouth, headache, excitability, nausea, heartburn, visual disturbances, restlessness, dizziness, drowsiness. *Warning:* If signs of drowsiness occur, deter your child from engaging in any potentially dangerous activity requiring alertness. May be addictive.

TUSSI-ORGANIDIN™*-DM* (℞). See TUSSI-ORGANIDIN™, above. This drug substitutes the antitussive dextromethorphan hydrobromide for codeine phosphate. Dosage for children, ½ to 1 teaspoon every 4 hours. Stomach upset is not included among side effects. This drug is not addictive. ☑ Not approved by the FDA.

√ *TUSS-ORNADE Liquid* (℞). For relief of cough and nasal congestion associated with the common cold. Carimiphen edisylate (antitussive), phenylpropanalamine hydrochloride (decongestant), alcohol (sedative and solvent). Do not use this drug if your child is sensitive to any of its ingredients; has bronchial asthma, coronary heart disease, or severe high blood pressure; or is receiving a MAO (monoamine oxidase) inhibitor or a CNS depressant. Your doctor may not prescribe this drug if your child has any type of cardiovascular disease, glaucoma, diabetes, thyroid disease, or if there is a therapeutic need for a productive cough. Dosage for children over 12 years of age, 2 teaspoons every 4 hours, up to 12 teaspoons in 24 hours; for children 6 to 12 years of age, 1 teaspoon every 4 hours, up to 6 teaspoons in 24 hours; for children 2 to 6 years of age, ½ teaspoon every 4 hours, up to 3 teaspoons in 24 hours. Do not use in children under 15 pounds or less than 3 months of age. For dosage for children 3 months to 2 years of age, consult your doctor. Common side effects: nausea, stomach upset, constipation or diarrhea, loss of appetite, chest pains, headache, clumsiness, palpitations, visual and urinary disorders, high or low blood pressure, nervousness, sleeplessness, dizziness, drowsiness. *Warning:* Should signs of drowsiness occur, deter your child from engaging in potentially dangerous activities requiring alertness. ☑ Not approved by the FDA.

TUSS-ORNADE Spansule Capsules (℞). Sustained-release. See TUSS-ORNADE Liquid in this section. Dosage for children over 12 years of age, 1 capsule every 24 hours. ☑ Not approved by the FDA.

VICKS DAYCARE CAPSULES (OTC). See VICKS DAYCARE LIQUID in this section. The capsule has no alcohol. Dosage for children 6 to 12 years of age, 1 capsule every 4 hours, up to 4 doses a day.

VICKS DAYCARE LIQUID (OTC). For relief of cold symptoms. Acetaminophen (analgesic, antipyretic), dextromethorphan hydrobromide (antitussive), phenylpropanolamine hydrochloride (decongestant), alcohol (sedative and solvent). Do not use without your doctor's approval if your child has diabetes, high blood pressure, heart or thyroid disease, high fever, or a persistent cough. Dosage for children 6 to 12 years of age, 1 tablespoon every 6 hours, up to 4 doses a day. The manufacturer reports no side effects at these dosages.

VICKS FORMULA 44 COUGH CONTROL DISC (OTC). To calm and quiet coughs and help soothe irritated throat. Dextromethorphan (antitussive), benzocaine (anesthetic), Special Vicks Medication (menthol, anethole, peppermint oil) (demulcent) in a dark brown sugar base. Do not use this preparation without your doctor's approval if your child has a high fever or a persistent cough. Dosage for children 4 to 12 years of age is 1 disc, dissolved in mouth, every 3 hours as needed. The manufacturer reports no significant side effects at this dosage.

VICKS FORMULA 44 COUGH MIXTURE (OTC). Syrup. For relief of cough and other symptoms of the common cold and other respiratory diseases. Dextromethorphan hydrobromide (antitussive), doxylamine succinate (antihistamine), sodium citrate (expectorant), alcohol (sedative and solvent) in a pleasant-tasting syrup. Do not use this mixture without your doctor's approval if your child has a high fever or a persistent cough. Dosage for children 6 to 12 years, 1 teaspoon every 4 hours as needed, up to 6 doses a day. The manufacturer reports no adverse side effects at this dosage.

√ *VICKS 44D DECONGESTANT COUGH MIXTURE* (OTC). For the relief of coughs, nasal congestion, and sore throat associated with the common cold, and for other respiratory discorders. Do not use without your doctor's approval if your child has a persistent cough, high blood pressure, diabetes, or heart or thyroid disease. Dosage for children 6 to 12 years of age, 1 teaspoon; for children 2 to 6 years of age, ½ teaspoon; repeat every 4 hours as needed, up to 6 doses per day.

VICKS HEADWAY CAPSULES (OTC). For relief of symptoms of the common cold. Phenylpropanolamine hydrochloride (decongestant), chlorpheniramine maleate (antihistamine). Do not use without approval of your doctor if your child has asthma, glaucoma, high blood pressure, heart or thyroid disease, difficulty urinating, or high fever, and do not use for more than 10 days. Dosage for children 6 to 12 years of age, 1 capsule every 4 hours, up to 6 doses a day. Common side effects: excitability and drowsiness. *Warning:* Should signs of drowsiness occur, deter your child from engaging in potentially dangerous activities requiring alertness.

VICKS HEADWAY TABLETS (OTC). See VICKS HEADWAY CAPSULES, above. Dosage for children 6 to 12 years of age, 1 tablet every 4 hours, up to 6 tablets a day.

4

Drugs to Treat Hay Fever and Other Allergies

I. DRUGS BASED ON ANTIHISTAMINES

Trade names
    See list of drugs in this section, page 108.

Ingredients
    Mainly antihistamines. For ingredients of individual drugs, see drugs in this section.

These drugs are used to
    Suppress the effects of allergens (substances which produce allergies).

How these drugs work
    The body's reaction to allergens is the production of histamines, chemicals which cause the symptoms of allergies: nasal congestion, watery and itchy eyes, a dry cough, sneezing (often violent and prolonged), mild itching, swell-

ing, and hives. Antihistamines suppress the action of histamines. Drugs in this section relieve the symptoms of hay fever and other allergies, not the causes.

The FDA has
    ☑ Approved these drugs.*
    ☐ Not approved these drugs.

These drugs are
    ☑ Effective.*
    ☐ Probably effective.
    ☐ Ineffective.

Dosage
See under individual drugs.
For a profile of antihistamines, see page 49.
Apply this profile to all antihistamine-containing drugs.

The drugs

√ *ACTIFED* (℞). Tablets and syrup. For relief of hay fever. Triprolidine hydrochloride (antihistamine), pseudoephedrine hydrochloride (decongestant). Pseudoephedrine hydrochloride should not be used, except on advice of your doctor, if your child has diabetes, glaucoma, heart or thyroid disease, or high blood pressure, or if your child is receiving MAO (monoamine oxidase) inhibitors, CNS depressants, drugs for asthma and other respiratory problems, or any one of several other drugs (consult your doctor). Common side effects of pseudoephedrine hydrochloride are nausea, vomiting, headache, difficulty in breathing and urinating, nervousness, restlessness, sleeplessness. Dosage for Actifed,

*See under individual drugs in this section for exceptions.

according to the manufacturer, "should be individualized according to the needs and responses of the patient." ☑ Not approved by the FDA.

√ *ALLEREST CHILDREN'S CHEWABLES* (OTC). For relief of hay fever, pollen allergies, upper respiratory allergies, allergic colds, sinusitis, and nasal passage congestion. Chlorpheniramine maleate (antihistamine), phenylpropanolamine hydrochloride (decongestant). Phenylpropanolamine should not be used except on advice of your doctor if your child has diabetes, heart disease, blood vessel disease, or if your child is receiving MAO (monoamine oxidase) inhibitors, CNS depressants, medicines for asthma or breathing problems, amphetamines, or guanethidine, or if your child is sensitive to either ingredient or chemicals related to phenylpropanolamine (consult your doctor). Common side effects of phenylpropanolamine: nervousness, restlessness, sleeplessness, dizziness, headache, nausea. Dosage for children 6 to 12 years of age, 2 tablets every 4 hours, up to 8 tablets in 24 hours; for children under 6 years of age, consult your doctor.

ALLEREST HEADACHE STRENGTH (OTC). See ALLEREST CHILDREN'S CHEWABLES, above. Dosage for children 6 to 12 years of age, 1 tablet every 4 hours, up to 4 tablets in 24 hours; for children under 6 years of age, consult your doctor.

ALLEREST TABLETS (OTC). See ALLEREST HEADACHE STRENGTH in this section. Same dosage.

ALLEREST TIMED RELEASE CAPSULES (OTC). See ALLEREST CHILDREN'S CHEWABLES, above. For dosage for children 12 years of age or over, consult your doctor.

√ *BENADRYL* (℞). Capsules, elixir, vials. For relief of hay fever, allergic conjunctivitis (inflammation of the membrane covering the front of the eyeball), and other allergic reactions. Diphenhydramine hydrochloride (antihistamine). Manufacturer recommends "dosage should be individualized according to the needs and the response of the patient." Suggested dosage, capsules and elixir, for children over 20 pounds of weight, 12.5 to 25.5 mg. 3 to 4 times daily, not to exceed 300 mg. per day. Parenteral (injectable) dose is prescribed when it is impractical to treat your child orally. Suggested dosage is 10 to 50 mg. intravenously or deeply intramuscularly; 100 mg. if required; to up 400 mg. daily.

√ *CHLOR-TRIMETON Allergy Syrup* (OTC). For relief of hay fever, allergic conjunctivitis (inflammation of the membrane covering the front of the eyeball), and other allergic reactions. Chlorpheniramine maleate (antihistamine), alcohol (sedative and solvent). Dosage for children 12 years of age or over, 2 teaspoons every 4 to 6 hours, up to 12 teaspoons in 24 hours; for children 6 through 11 years of age, 1 teaspoon every 4 to 6 hours, up to 6 teaspoons in 24 hours; for children under 6 years of age, consult your physician. ☑ Not approved by the FDA.

CHLOR-TRIMETON Allergy Tablets (OTC). See CHLOR-TRIMETON Allergy Syrup, above. For children 12 years of age or over, 1 tablet every 4 to 6 hours, up to 6 tablets in 24 hours; for children 6 to 11 years of age, ½ tablet every 4 to 6 hours, up to 3 tablets in 24 hours; for children under 6 years of age, consult your doctor.

CHLOR-TRIMETON Long-Acting Allergy REPETABS Tablets (OTC). For relief, for up to 12 hours, of hay fever, allergic conjunctivitis (inflammation of the membrane covering the front of the eyeball), and other allergic reactions. Chlorpheniramine maleate (antihistamine). Dosage for children 12 years of age or over, 1 tablet in the morning and 1 at night, up to 3 tablets a day; for children under 12 years of age, consult your doctor.

√ *CONTAC* (OTC). For relief of hay fever, as well as nasal congestion due to the common cold and sinusitis. See CONTAC Continuous Action Decongestant Capsules, page 73.

√ *CORICIDIN* (OTC). Tablets. For relief of symptoms of hay fever, as well as the common cold. See CORICIDIN, page 75.

√ *DIMETANE EXPECTORANT* (℞). Syrup. For treatment of allergies as well as relief of coughing. Bromopheniramine maleate (antihistamine), guaifenesin (expectorant), phenylephrine hydrochloride (decongestant), phenylpropanolamine hydrochloride (decongestant). Do not use if your child is sensitive to any of these ingredients. Side effects of guaifenesin are stomach pain, nausea, vomiting, diarrhea, and drowsiness. Do not use phenylephrine hydrochloride without your doctor's approval if your child has heart or blood vessel disorders or high blood pressure, or is taking MAO (monoamine oxidase) inhibitors, guanethidine, or other medicines to lower blood pressure, alpha blockers (alpha-adrenergic blocking agents), or tricyclic antidepressants. Side effects of phenylephrine hydrochloride include restlessness, nervousness, dizziness, weakness, paleness, trouble breathing, chest pains, or discomfort. For a description of phenylpropanolamine hydrochloride, see ALLEREST CHILDREN'S CHEWABLES in this section. Dosage for children, ½ to 1 teaspoon 3 to 4 times a day. ☑ Not approved by the FDA.

111

√ *DIMETAPP ELIXIR* (℞). Grape-flavored. For relief of hay fever, allergies, coughs. Bromopheniramine maleate (antihistamine), phenylephrine hydrochloride (decongestant), phenylpropanolamine hydrochloride (decongestant), alcohol (sedative and solvent). See DIMETANE EXPECTORANT in this section. Dosage for children 4 to 12 years of age, 1 teaspoon 2 to 4 times daily; for children 2 to 4 years of age, ¾ teaspoon 2 to 4 times daily; for children 7 months to 2 years of age, ½ teaspoon 3 to 4 times daily; for children 1 month to 6 months, ¼ teaspoon 3 to 4 times daily. ☑ Not approved by the FDA. This drug is ☑ probably effective, as classified by the FDA.

DIMETAPP EXTENTABS (℞). Sustained-release tablet version of Dimetapp Elixir. Does not contain alcohol. For children 12 years of age or over, 1 tablet morning and evening, or 3 tablets a day. ☑ Not approved by the FDA. This drug is ☑ probably effective, as classified by the FDA.

√ *DRIXORAL Sustained-Action Tablets* (℞). For the relief of nasal and upper respiratory congestion associated with allergies. Dexbromopheniramine maleate (antihistamine), pseudoephedrine sulfate (decongestant). For a description of pseudoephedrine, see under ACTIFED in this section. Dosage for children under 12 years of age, 1 tablet in the morning and 1 at bedtime; or 1 tablet every 8 hours in exceptional cases.

√ *NOVAHISTINE ELIXIR* (OTC). For relief of nasal and upper respiratory congestion associated with allergies. See NOVAHISTINE ELIXIR, page 86.

√ *ORNADE 2 LIQUID FOR CHILDREN* (OTC). For relief of nasal congestion associated with allergies. See ORNADE 2 LIQUID FOR CHILDREN, page 87.

PB Z (℞). Elixir, tablets, sustained-release tablets. For the treatment of many types of allergies. Tripelennamine (antihistamine). Dosage for children and infants, 5 mg. per kilogram (about 2.2 lb.) of weight, up to 300 mg. each 24 hours, divided into 6 to 8 doses.

√ *PERIACTIN SYRUP* (℞). For relief of hay fever, allergic conjunctivitis (inflammation of the membrane covering the front of the eyeball), hives, and other allergic reactions. Cyproheptacline (antihistamine). Dosage for children 7 to 14 years of age, 2 teaspoons 2 or 3 times daily, up to 4 teaspoons if needed; for children 2 to 6 years of age, 1 teaspoon 2 to 3 times a day, up to 6 teaspoons if needed.

√ *PHENERGAN* (℞). Tablets, syrup, rectal suppositories. For relief of hay fever and a wide variety of allergic reactions. Promethazine hydrochloride (antihistamine). Oral dosage for children, 25 mg. before bedtime or 6.25 to 12.5 mg. 3 times a day; rectal dosage for children, 25 mg., repeated 2 hours later if needed.

POLARAMINE (℞). Tablets, syrup. For relief of hay fever and a wide variety of allergic reactions. Dexchlorpheniramine maleate (antihistamine). Dosage for Polaramine, according to the manufacturer, "should be individualized according to the needs and responses of the patient." Suggested dosage: tablets, for children 12 years of age or over, 1 tablet every 4 to 6 hours; for children 6 through 11 years of age, ½ tablet every 4 to 6 hours; for children 2 to 6 years of age, ¼ tablet every 4 to 6 hours; syrup, for children 12 years of age or older, 1 teaspoon every 4 to 6 hours; for children 6 through 11 years of age, ¼ teaspoon every 4 to 6 hours; for children 2 to 5 years of age, ¼ teaspoon every 4 to 6 hours.

√ *TELDRIN Timed-Release Energy Capsules* (OTC). For up to 12 hours' relief from symptoms of hay fever and other respiratory allergies. Chlorpheniramine maleate (antihistamine). Dosage for Teldrin, according to the manufacturer, "should be individualized according to the needs and responses of the patient." Suggested dosage for children over 12 years of age, 1 tablet in morning and 1 in evening; for children under 12 years of age, consult your doctor.

II. DRUGS BASED ON ADRENOCORTICOIDS (Corticosteroids)

Trade names
See list of drugs in this section, page 118.

Ingredients
Adrenocorticoids are cortisonelike drugs belonging to the chemical family of steroids.

Warning: External steroid medicines bypass the body's internal hormone production. This leads to various hormonal inbalances. The pituitary gland which, in part, regulates the growth process, may be thrown off balance. Thyroid function may be disturbed. Fluid may be retained as a direct side effect of steroid medicines. There is even the possibility of disturbance of brain function.

These drugs are used to
Treat a wide range of allergies as well as other diseases.

How these drugs work
Reduce swelling, redness, itching, and reactions from allergens.

The FDA has
☑ Approved these drugs.
☐ Not approved these drugs.

These drugs are
- ☑ Effective.
- ☐ Probably effective.
- ☐ Ineffective.

These drugs should not be used under the following conditions
- Fungal infections involving the entire system.

Your doctor may not approve use of these drugs under the following conditions
If your child has:
- Stomach or intestinal disorders.
- Glaucoma.
- Herpes simplex of the eye.
- Tuberculosis (past or present).
- Kidney or liver disease.
- Diabetes.
- Heart disease.
- High cholesterol levels.
- High blood pressure.
- Hypothyroidism.
- Myasthenia gravis (See page 39).
- Bone disease.

The use of the following drugs decreases the effectiveness of these drugs
- Phenytoin, phenobarbital, ephedrine, rifampin.

How these drugs interact with other drugs
Do not use these drugs with the following drugs:
- Oral blood thinners (anticoagulants).
- Insulin.
- Oral diabetes medicines.
- Most diuretics.

- Cardiac glycosides.
- Tetracycline.
- Arthritis drugs, and other drugs to reduce inflammation.
- Digitalis.
- Antihypertiensives (drugs to lower blood pressure).
- Amphotericin B.
- Somatropin.
- Drugs for skin tests and immunizations, especially smallpox.

How these drugs are supplied

See under individual drugs in this section.

Dosage

See under individual drugs in this section.

Common side effects

- Muscle pain, cramps, or weakness.
- Pains in back or ribs.
- Suppressed growth.
- Osteoporosis (decrease in bone density).
- Fatigue.
- Nausea, vomiting.
- Indigestion.
- Stomach pain.
- Appetite increase.
- Weight gain.
- Fatty deposits in face, neck, and abdomen.
- Impaired wound healing.
- Increased chance of infection.
- Increased chance of bruising.
- Fever.
- Sore throat.
- Skin alterations, including acne.

- Visual problems.
- Swelling of legs, feet, and other parts of the body.
- Restlessness.
- Nervousness.
- Sleeplessness.
- Mood swings.
- Depression.
- Unnatural "highs" (euphoria).
- Loss of potassium.
- Retention of sodium and water.
- Irregular heartbeat.
- High blood pressure.

Effects of long-term use
Some side effects are related to length of treatment.

After-use effects
- Loss of appetite.
- Significant weight loss.
- Fatigue.
- Shortness of breath.
- Dizziness.
- Nausea, vomiting.
- Fever.
- Pains in the back or abdomen.

The drugs

DELTASONE (℞). Tablets. For treatment of allergies and a wide range of inflammatory diseases. Prednisone. Dosage is individualized; consult your doctor.

√ *MEDROL* (℞). Tablets. For the treatment of allergies and a wide range of inflammatory diseases. Methylprednisolone. Dosage is individualized; consult your doctor.

METICORTEN (℞). See DELTASONE in this section.

√ *ORASONE* (℞). See DELTASONE in this section.

√ *STERAPRED* (℞). See DELTASONE in this section.

5

Drugs to Treat Asthma

Trade names
    See list of drugs in this section, page 122.

Ingredients
    See under *How these drugs work* and under individual drugs in this section.

These drugs are used to
    Help relieve symptoms of bronchial asthma: wheezing, difficulty of breathing, cough.

How these drugs work
    This is how the classes of drugs in antiasthmatic medicines act:
    Andrenergic bronchodilators (sympathomimetic agents): act to relax the smooth bronchial muscle. The contraction of this muscle narrows the breathing passage to the lungs. Examples: ephedrine and epinephrine.
    Corticosteroids: act to reduce the swelling and inflammation of the walls of the bronchi, which shrink the breathing passage. Example: dexamethasone sodium phosphate.

Xanthines: act to relax the smooth bronchial muscle. See ANDRENERGIC BRONCHODILATORS in this section.

Some drugs in these classes are used in combination with each other, and with expectorants and decongestants, which help remove thick mucus plugs which block the breathing passage. Sedatives sometimes are added to the combinations.

The FDA has
 ☑ Approved these drugs.*
 ☐ Not approved these drugs.

The drugs

ALUPENT (℞). Tablets, syrup. For treatment of bronchial asthma, bronchitis, and emphysema. Metaproterenol sulfate (andrenergic bronchodilator). Do not use this drug if your child has an irregular heartbeat associated with tachycardia. Your doctor may not prescribe this drug if your child is sensitive to this drug or other sympathomimetic amines or has heart disease, high blood pressure, diabetes, or hypertension, or if your child is receiving other asthma drugs, drugs to relieve breathing problems, propranolol, or amphetamines. The effectiveness of this drug is decreased by nonselective beta blockers. Dosage for children 9 to 12 years of age or over 60 pounds of body weight, 20 mg. or 2 teaspoons 3 or 4 times a day; for children 6 to 9 years of age or under 60 pounds, 10 mg. or 1 teaspoon 3 or 4 times a day. Common side effects are nausea, vomiting, nervousness, restlessness, high blood pressure, irregular heartbeat, palpitations, bad taste in the mouth.

AMINOPHYLLIN (℞). Tablets, ampules. For treatment of bronchial asthma, bronchitis, and emphysema. Aminophyl-

*See under individual drugs in this section for exceptions.

line (xanthine). Do not use this drug if your child is sensitive to aminophylline or theophylline. Your doctor may not prescribe this drug if your child has or has had a stomach ulcer; liver, kidney, or heart disease; hyperthyroidism; or high blood pressure. Epinephrine and other sympathomimetic agents, other xanthines, and the antibiotics erythromycin, clindamycin, lincomycin, and troleoandomycin received concurrently with Aminophyllin increase the risk of toxicity. The effectiveness of this drug is decreased by propranolol; and this drug decreases the effectiveness of lithium. Dosage: tablets for children with acute bronchial asthma, 12 mg. per kilogram (about 2.2 lb.) of body weight every 24 hours in 4 divided doses; for intramuscular injection, consult your doctor. Common side effects: irritability, nervousness, restlessness, sleeplessness, nausea, vomiting, stomach pain, headache, bitter aftertaste, hives; when injected, side effects also include an increase in blood pressure and rash.

√ *AMODRINE* (OTC, ℞ in some states). For relief of bronchial asthma symptoms (wheezing, shortness of breath). Ephedrine hydrochloride, racemic (adrenergic bronchodilator), aminophylline (xanthine), and phenobarbital (sedative). For a profile of ephedrine, see ACTIFED, page 108; for a profile of aminophylline, see AMINOPHYLLIN in this section; and for a profile of phenobarbital, see page 227. Use this drug only if your doctor tells you your child has asthma. Prescription drug is ☑not approved by the FDA.

BECLOVANT (℞). Metered-dose inhalator. For treatment of chronic asthma. Beclomethasone diproprionate (corticosteroid). For a profile of corticosteroid used to treat asthma, see RESPIHALER DECADRON PHOSPHATE in this section. Dosage for children 6 to 12 years of age, 1 inhalation to 2 inhalations 3 or 4 times a day, up to 10 inhalations in 24 hours.

BRETHINE (℞). Tablets. For treatment of bronchial asthma. Terbutaline sulfate (an andrenergic bronchodilator). Do not use this drug if your child is sensitive to it or to other sympathomimetic agents. Your doctor may not prescribe this drug if your child has heart disease, high blood pressure diabetes, seizures (past or present), or hyperthyroidism; or if your child is receiving asthma drugs, other drugs to relieve breathing difficulties, propanolol, or amphetamines. Dosage for children 12 to 15 years of age, 2.5 mg. 3 times a day during waking hours, up to 7.5 mg. in 24 hours. Common side effects: nervousness, restlessness, tremors.

BRICANYL (℞). Tablets. See BRETHINE, above.

BRONDECON (℞). Elixir. For treatment of bronchial asthma and other chronic obstructive pulmonary diseases. Oxytriphylline (xanthine), guaifenesin (expectorant). For a profile of a xanthine, see AMINOPHYLLIN in this section. Dosage for children 2 to 12 years, 1 teaspoon for every 60 pounds of body weight 4 times a day, or as your doctor prescribes.

√ *BRONITIN* (OTC). Tablets. For relief of bronchial asthma symptoms (wheezing, shortness of breath, and congestion). Ephedrine hydrochloride (adrenergic bronchodilator), pyrilamine maleate (antihistamine), guaifenesin (expectorant). For a profile of ephedrine hydrochloride, see ACTIFED, page 108. Guaifenesin is a drug which can be used in almost all conditions except sensitivity to it and has no significant drug interactions or common side effects. Dosage for children 6 to 12 years of age, ½ tablet every 3 or 4 hours, up to 5 doses in 24 hours; for children under 6 years of age, consult your doctor.

BRONITON MIST (OTC). Aerosol, for inhalation only. For relief of bronchial asthma symptoms (wheezing, shortness of breath). Epinephrine bitartrate (adrenergic bronchodilator). Do not use without approval of your doctor if your child has high blood pressure, diabetes, or heart or thyroid disease. This drug reacts adversely with a wide variety of drugs; consult your doctor. Dosage: for children 6 years of age or over, 1 inhalation repeated after 1 minute if no relief occurs, no more than 2 inhalations in 4 hours; for children under 6 years of age, consult your doctor. Common side effect: dryness of mouth.

√ *BRONKAID MIST* (OTC). Aerosol, for inhalation only. Epinephrine (adrenergic bronchodilator). See BRONITIN MIST in this section.

√ *BRONKAID TABLETS* (OTC). For relief of bronchial asthma symptoms and congestion. Ephedrine sulfate (adrenergic bronchodilator), guaifenesin (expectorant), theophylline (xanthine). For a profile of ephedrine, see ACTIFED, page 108. For a profile of guaifenesin, see BRONITIN in this section. For a profile of xanthines, see AMINOPHYLLIN in this section. Dosage: same as BRONITIN in this section.

BRONKOLIXIR (OTC). Cherry-flavored elixir. Ingredients same as for BRONKOTABS, below, plus alcohol (sedative, solvent). Dosage for children over 6 years of age, 1 teaspoon every 3 or 4 hours, 4 times daily; for children under 6 years of age, consult your doctor.

√ *BRONKOTABS* (OTC). Tablets. For treatment of bronchial asthma, as indicated by the actions of the following ingredients: ephedrine sulfate (adrenergic bronchodilator), guaifenesin (expectorant), theophylline (xanthine), and phenobarbital (sedative). For a profile of ephedrine, see ACTIFED, page 108. For profiles of guaifenesin, xanthines, and phenobarbital, see pages 124, 122, and 227, respectively. Dosage for children over 6 years of age, ½ tablet every 3 to 4 hours, 4 or 5 times a day; for children under 6 years of age, consult your doctor. May be addictive.

CHOLEDYL (R). Elixir. Oxtriphylline (xanthine). For a profile of a xanthine, see AMINOPHYLLIN in this section. Dosage for children 2 to 12 years of age: 1 teaspoon per 60 pounds of body weight, 4 times a day.

√ *CHOLEDYL PEDIATRIC SYRUP* (R). For treatment of acute bronchial asthma. Oxtriphylline (xanthine). For a profile of a xanthine, see AMINOPHYLLIN in this section. Dosage is determined by body weight; consult your doctor.

ELIXOPHYLLIN (R). Capsules, sustained-release capsules, elixir. For treatment of acute bronchial asthma. Theophylline (xanthine). For a profile of a xanthine, see AMINOPHYLLIN in this section. Dosage is determined by body weight; consult your doctor.

INTAL (R). Capsules for inhalation only. Use as an adjunct in treatment of severe bronchial asthma to prevent attacks; do not use during attacks. Cromoleyn sodium. Do not use if your child is sensitive to this drug or has a liver or kidney disorder. Dosage for children over 5 years of age, 20 mg. inhaled 4 times a day at regular intervals. Common side effects: cough, hoarseness, throat irritation, trouble swallowing, stuffy nose, watery eyes, swelling of lips and eyes, nausea, vomiting, dizziness, headache, urinary difficulties, rash, hives, joint swelling and pain, chest tightness, breathing difficulties.

ISUPREL (R). Metered dose inhaler. For bronchospasms associated with acute and bronchial asthma. Isoproterenol hydrochloride (andrenergic bronchodilator). Do not use this drug if your child is sensitive to it or to drugs related to it (consult your doctor) or has an irregular heartbeat associated with tachycardia. Your doctor may not prescribe this drug if your child has any heart disease, blood vessel disease, high blood pressure, diabetes, or hyperthyroidism, or if your child is receiving other asthma drugs, drugs for breathing problems, propranolol, or amphetamines. Dosage for children: for acute episodes, 1 inhalation followed by another in 1 minute if needed, up to 5 doses a day; for chronic conditions, 1 inhalation to 2 inhalations not less than 3 or 4 hours apart. Common side effects: dryness of mouth, chest pain, irregular heartbeat, nervousness, restlessness, sleeplessness, nausea, vomiting, trembling, dizziness, light-headedness, flushing, redness of face and skin.

√ MARAX (℞). Tablets, syrup. For control of bronchospasms. Ephedrine sulfate (adrenergic bronchodilator), theophylline (xanthine), and hydroxyzine hydrochloride (sedative). For a profile of ephedrine, see ACTIFED, page 108. For a profile of a xanthine, see AMINOPHYLLIN in this section. For a profile of hydroxyzine hydrochloride, see ATARAX, page 50. Dosage for children 2 to 5 years of age, ½ to 1 teaspoon syrup 3 or 4 times a day; for children over 5 years of age, ½ tablet 2 to 4 times a day, at least 4 hours between doses, or 1 teaspoon 3 to 4 times a day. This drug is ☑ not approved by the FDA and is classified by the FDA as ☑ probably effective.

√ PRIMATINE MIST (OTC). Aerosol for inhalation. For the relief of acute paroxysms of bronchial asthma. Epinephrine bitartrate (andrenergic bronchodilator). For a profile of epinephrine, see BRONITIN MIST in this section. Dosage for children 1 inhalation, followed by another in 1 minute if needed; do not repeat for at least 4 hours. Note: OTC drugs should not be used in combination with prescription medications unless carefully monitored.

127

√ *PRIMATINE TABLETS "M"* (OTC). For relief and control of bronchial asthma and associated hay fever. Theophylline (xanthine), ephedrine hydrochloride (andrenergic bronchodilator), pyrilamine maleate (antihistamine). For profile of a xanthine, see AMINOPHYLLIN in this section. For a profile of ephedrine, see ACTIFED, page 108. For a profile of antihistamines, see page 49. Dosage for children 6 to 12 years of age, ½ to 1 tablet to start; then ½ tablet every 4 hours, up to 6 tablets in 24 hours. See Note on OTC drugs, page 127.

PRIMATINE TABLETS "P" (OTC). Ingredients same as for PRIMATINE TABLETS "M," above, except that pyrilamine maleate is replaced by phenobarbital. For a profile of phenobarbital, see page 227. See Note on OTC drugs, page 127.

QUADRINAL (℞). Tablets, suspension. For chronic asthma characterized by hard-to-loosen mucus and bronchospasm; it is also used in the treatment of chronic bronchitis and pulmonary emphysema. Ephedrine hydrochloride (andrenergic bronchodilator), theophylline calcium salicylate (xanthine), phenobarbital (sedative), potassium iodide (expectorant). For a profile of ephedrine, see ACTIFED, page 108. For a profile of a xanthine, see AMINOPHYLLIN in this section. For a profile of phenobarbital, see page 227. Do not use a potassium iodide medicine without approval of your doctor if your child has kidney disease or heart disease, untreated hyperthyroidism, tuberculosis, or underactive adrenals, or is receiving triamterene, spironolactone, lithium, or drugs containing potassium. Common side effects of potassium iodide: nausea, vomiting, stomach pains, diarrhea, skin rash, irregular heartbeat, fever, fatigue, heavy and weak feeling in legs, numbness and tingling in hands or feet, swelling of neck or throat, confusion. Quadrinal dosage for children 6 to 12 years of age, ½ tablet or 1 teaspoon 3 times a day; for children under 6 years of age, consult your doctor. This drug is ☑ not approved by the FDA.

√ *QUIBRON* (℞). Capsules, liquid, For treatment of bronchospasms. Theophylline (xanthine) and guaifenesin (expectorant). For a profile of xanthines, see AMINOPHYLLIN in this section. For a profile of guaifenesin, see BRONITIN in this section. Dosage for children is determined by body weight; consult your doctor.

RESPIHALER DECADRON PHOSPHATE (℞). Metered dose inhaler. For treatment of bronchial asthma. Dexamethasone sodium phosphate (corticosteroid). Do not use this drug if your child is sensitive to this drug or has a fungal infection or an infection of nose, throat, or sinuses. Dosage for children: 2 inhalations 3 or 4 times a day, up to 8 inhalations a day. Common side effects: nasal dryness and irritation, loss of sense of smell, nosebleeds, shortness of breath, trouble breathing.

√ *SUSPENSION TEDRAL ELIXIR* (OTC). For treatment of symptoms of bronchial asthma (wheezing, shortness of breath). Theophylline (xanthine), ephedrine hydrochloride (adrenergic bronchodilator), phenobarbital (sedative), alcohol (sedative and solvent). For profile of a xanthine, see AMINOPHYLLIN in this section. For a profile of ephedrine, see ACTIFED, page 108. For a profile of phenobarbital, see page 227. Dosage for children: 1 teaspoon per 60 lb. of body weight every 4 to 6 hours; for children under 2 years of age, consult your doctor.

TEDRAL TABLETS (OTC). Ingredients same as for SUSPENSION TEDRAL ELIXIR, above, except that alcohol is omitted. Dosage for children over 60 pounds, ½ to 1 tablet every 4 hours. ☑ Not approved by the FDA.

TEDRAL 8A (℞). Sustained-action tablets. Ingredients same as for TEDRAL TABLETS in this section, except for sustained-action formulation. For children 12 years of age or over, 1 tablet on waking, another 12 hours later. ☑ Not approved by the FDA.

TEDRAL EXPECTORANT (℞). Tablets. Ingredients same as for TEDRAL TABLETS in this section, except that guaifenesin (expectorant) is added. For a profile of guaifenesin, see BRONITIN in this section. For children 12 or over, 1 tablet every 4 hours. ☑ Not approved by the FDA.

TEDRAL-25 (℞). Ingredients same as for TEDRAL TABLETS in this section, except for the amounts of ingredients. Dosage for children 6 to 12 years of age, ½ tablet every 4 hours. ☑ Not approved by the FDA.

VANCERIL (℞). See BECLOVANT in this section.

6

Drugs to Treat Constipation, Diarrhea, and Other Gastrointestinal Disorders

DRUGS TO TREAT CONSTIPATION

Trade names
See list of drugs in this section, page 133.

Ingredients
See under *How these drugs work* and under individual drugs in this section.

These drugs are used to
Treat constipation, a disorder in which the bowels move with less than normal frequency and ease.

How these drugs work
This is how the classes of drugs in constipation medicines act:
Bulk-forming laxatives—facilitate bowel movement by increasing the size of the stools. Example: psyllium seeds.

131

Lubricant laxatives—facilitate bowel movement by softening the contents of the intestine. Example: mineral oil.

Saline laxatives—facilitate bowel movement by increasing the amount of water in the colon. These laxatives are characterized by rapid action. Example: Epsom salts (magnesium sulfate).

Stimulant laxatives—facilitate bowel movement by stimulating the muscular action of the intestine that forces the stool downward (peristalsis). Example: castor oil.

Some drugs are used by themselves in constipation medicines; other constipation medicines combine two or more constipation drugs.

The FDA has
- ☑ Not disapproved these drugs.*
- ☐ Disapproved these drugs.

These drugs are
- ☑ Effective.**
- ☐ Probably effective.
- ☐ Ineffective.

These drugs should not be used under the following conditions
- If your child experiences pains in the stomach or abdomen, bloating, cramping, nausea, vomiting, or high fever. Consult your doctor.
- If your child has been receiving laxatives regularly for more than 1 week to 2 weeks without approval of

*Most constipation drugs are OTC.

**But overuse can make constipation worse or even induce constipation. Drugs vary in speed of action.

your doctor. *Caution:* Laxatives used over long periods of time may result in dependence on these drugs.

- See under individual drugs in this section.

The drugs

√ *AGORAL Marshmallow* (OTC). Marshmallow-flavored emulsion. Ingredients same as for AGORAL Plain, below, except for the flavor and phenophthalein (stimulant laxative). Do not use if your doctor regards the action of phenophthalein as too harsh for your child, or if your child is sensitive to that drug. Do not use any stimulant laxative without approval of your physician if your child has gastrointestinal disorders, the laxative habit, appendicitis or possible appendicitis, inflamed bowel, diabetes, congestive heart disease, kidney disease, high blood pressure, or undiagnosed rectal bleeding, or if your child is receiving other laxatives, blood thinners (anticoagulants), antacids, antibiotics, or medicines containing digitalis. Dosage for children over 6 years of age, 1 teaspoon to 2 teaspoons taken in the same way as Agoral Plain. Side effects are not common, but your child may experience cramps, diarrhea, belching, nausea, or skin rash.

√ *AGORAL Plain* (OTC). Emulsion. Mineral oil (lubricant laxative), glycerin (stimulant laxative), agar, tragacanth, and acacia (bulk-forming laxatives), egg albumin (emulsifier). For a profile of stimulant laxatives, see AGORAL Marshmallow, above. Do not use any lubricant laxative without your doctor's approval if your child has gastrointestinal disorders, the laxative habit, appendicitis or possible appendicitis, inflamed bowel, diabetes, congestive heart disease, or undiagnosed rectal bleeding, or if your child is receiving other laxatives, blood thinners (anticoagulants), medicines containing digitalis, or vitamins A, D, E, or K. Lubricant laxatives may reduce the effectiveness of other medicines taken within 2 hours of the laxative dose. Common side effects of some lubricant laxatives are skin rash, nausea, stomach cramps, and throat irritation when taken orally. Do not use any bulk-forming laxative without your doctor's approval if your child has any of the diseases listed previously under this item, or if your child is receiving other laxatives, blood thinners (anticoagulants), medicines containing digitalis, or aspirin or other salicylates. Bulk-forming laxatives may reduce the effectiveness of other medicines taken within 2 hours of the laxative dose. If your child is on a low-salt, low-sugar, or low-carbohydrate diet, consult your doctor before using bulk-forming laxatives, since they contain large amounts of salt, sugar, and carbohydrates. There are no common side effects associated with bulk-forming laxatives. Dosage for children over 6 years of age, 2 to 4 teaspoons, taken at bedtime (unless your doctor advises otherwise), alone or with any food or drink in which it can be mixed. No adverse side effects reported by the manufacturer.

√ *AGORAL Raspberry* (OTC). Raspberry-flavored emulsion. See AGORAL Marshmallow in this section.

√ *COLACE* (OTC). Capsules. Dioctyl sodium sulfosuccinate (docusate sodium) (lubricant laxative). For a profile of lubricant laxatives, see AGORAL Plain in this section. Dosage for children 6 to 12 years of age, 40 to 120 mg. per day as needed; for children 3 to 6 years of age, 20 to 60 mg.; for children under 3 years of age, 10 to 40 mg.

√ *COLACE Liquid* (OTC). See COLACE in this section. To mask bitter taste, give this drug in milk, fruit juice, or infant formula. For use in enemas, add 5 to 10 ml. to retention or flushing enema.

√ *COLACE Syrup* (OTC). See COLACE in this section.

√ *COMFOLAX* (OTC). Capsules. Dioctyl sodium sulfosucci-nate (docusate sodium) (lubricant laxative). For a profile of lubricant laxatives, see AGORAL Plain in this section. Dosage for children 12 years of age or over, 1 capsule or 2 capsules daily, increased to 2 capsules twice daily in stubborn cases.

COMFOLAX-plus (OTC). Capsules. Ingredients same as for COMFOLAX, above, plus casanthranol (stimulant laxative). For a profile of stimulant laxatives, see AGORAL Marshmal-low in this section. Dosage for children over 12 years of age, 1 capsule or 2 capsules at bedtime for 1 day or 2 days, then 1 capsule a day as needed.

DIALOSE (OTC). Capsules. Dioctyl sodium sulfosuccinate (docusate sodium) (lubricant laxative). For a profile of lubricant laxatives, see AGORAL Plain in this section. Dosage for children 6 years of age or over, 1 capsule at bedtime, or as directed by your doctor; for children under 6 years of age, consult your doctor.

DORBANTYL (OTC). Capsules. Danthron (stimulant) and dioctyl sodium sulfosuccinate (docusate sodium) (lubricant laxative). For profiles of stimulant and lubricant laxatives, see AGORAL Marshmallow and AGORAL Plain respectively, in this section. Dosage for children 6 to 12 years of age, 1 capsule at bedtime.

DOXIDAN (OTC). See DORBANTYL in this section.

DOXINATE (OTC). Capsules. See COMFOLAX in this section. Dosage for children over 6 years of age, 60 to 120 mg. a day.

DOXINATE Solution (OTC). Ingredients same as for DOXI-NATE in this section, plus alcohol (sedative and solvent).

Dosage for children 6 to 12 years of age, ½ to 1 teaspoon a day (may be mixed with milk or juice); for children 3 to 6 years of age, ⅕ to ⅖ teaspoon a day (may be mixed with milk or juice).

EFFERSYLLIUM Powder (OTC). Psyllium hydrocolloid (bulk-forming laxative). For a profile of bulk-forming laxatives, see AGORAL Plain in this section. Dosage for children over 6 years of age, 1 level teaspoon or ½ packet in 4 ounces of water at bedtime.

EX-LAX Unflavored or Chocolate Tablets or Chewable Tablets (OTC). Yellow phenophthalein (stimulant laxative). For a profile of stimulant laxatives, see AGORAL Marshmallow in this section. Dosage for children over 6 years of age, 1 tablet with water, preferably at bedtime.

FLEET ENEMA (OTC). Sodium phosphate, sodium biphosphate (saline laxatives). Do not use saline laxatives without your doctor's approval if your child has gastrointestinal disorders, the laxative habit, appendicitis or possible appendicitis, inflamed bowel, diabetes, congestive heart disease, kidney disease, or undiagnosed rectal bleeding, or if your child is receiving other laxatives, blood thinners (anticoagulants), medicines containing digitalis, medicines to treat diabetes or emotional conditions, isoniazid, and tetracyclines; or if your child is on a low-sodium diet. Dosage for children over 2 years of age, 2 fluid ounces.

FLEET MINERAL OIL ENEMA (OTC). Mineral oil (lubricant laxative). For a profile of lubricant laxatives, see AGORAL Plain in this section. Dosage for children over 2 years of age, 1 fluid ounce to 2 fluid ounces.

√ *GLYCERIN PEDIATRIC SUPPOSITORIES* (OTC). Glycerin (stimulant laxative), emulsified and stiffened with sodium stearate. For a profile of stimulant laxatives, see AGORAL Marshmallow in this section. Dosage for children, 1 suppository inserted and retained for 15 minutes.

√ *MALTSUPEX* (OTC). Tablets. Malt soup extract (bulk-forming laxative). For a profile of bulk-forming laxatives, see AGORAL Plain in this section. For children, 1 teaspoon to 2 teaspoons in milk or on cereal 1 time or 2 times a day, for infants over 1 month of age, bottle-fed, ½ teaspoon to 2 teaspoons a day added to feeding (use 1 teaspoon to 2 teaspoons to prevent constipation); breast-fed, 1 teaspoon to 2 teaspoons in 2 to 4 ounces of water or juice before feedings, 1 or 2 times a day.

MILK OF MAGNESIA (OTC). Suspension. Magnesium hydroxide (saline laxative). For a profile of saline laxatives, see FLEET ENEMA in this section. For children over 1 year of age, 1 teaspoon a day; for children under 1 year of age, consult your doctor.

√ *MINERAL OIL* (OTC). Liquid. Mineral oil (lubricant laxative). For a profile of lubricant laxatives, see AGORAL Plain in this section. Dosage for children: 1 teaspoon to 3 teaspoons at bedtime.

MITROLAN Chewable Tablets (OTC). Calcium polycarbophil (bulk-forming laxative). For a profile of bulk-forming laxatives, see AGORAL Plain in this section. Dosage for children 6 to 11 years of age, 1 tablet 3 times a day, or as needed, up to 6 tablets in 24 hours; for children 3 to 5 years of age, 1 tablet 2 times a day, or as needed, up to 3 tablets in 24 hours; tablets are to be chewed before swallowing.

MODANE Liquid (OTC). Ingredients same as for MODANE Tablets in this section, plus alcohol (sedative and solvent). Dosage for children 6 to 12 years of age, 1 teaspoon with supper; for children 1 year to 6 years of age, ¼ to 1 tea-spoon with supper; for children 6 to 12 months of age ⅕ to ¼ teaspoon with supper.

MODANE Tablets (OTC). Danthron (stimulant laxative). For a profile of stimulant laxatives, see AGORAL Marshmallow in this section. Dosage for children 6 to 12 years of age, 37.5 ms. with supper.

PERDIEM (OTC). Granules. Psyllium (bulk-forming laxa-tive), senna (stimulant laxative). For profiles of bulk-forming and stimulant laxatives, see AGORAL Plain and AGORAL Marshmallow, respectively, in this section. Dosage for children 7 to 11 years of age, 1 rounded teaspoon 1 time or 2 times a day.

PERI-COLACE Syrup (OTC). Casanthranol (stimulant laxa-tive), dioctyl sodium sulfosuccinate (docusate sodium) (lubricant laxative). For profiles of stimulant and lubricant laxatives, see AGORAL Marshmallow and AGORAL Plain, respectively, in this section. Dosage for children: 1 tea-spoon to 3 teaspoons at bedtime.

PHOSPHO-SODA (OTC). Solution. Sodium phosphate, sodium biphosphate (saline laxatives). For a profile of saline laxatives, see FLEET ENEMA in this section. Dosage for chil-dren over 10 years of age, 2 teaspoons; for children 5 to 10 years of age, 1 teaspoon; Phospho-Soda doses are mixed with 4 ounces of cold water and are followed by 8 ounces of cold water; this drug is taken on rising, or at least 30 minutes before a meal, or at bedtime.

RECTALAD ENEMA (OTC). Glycerin, soft soap (stimulant laxatives), dioctyl potassium sulfosuccinate (docusate po-tassium) (lubricant laxative). For profiles of stimulant and lubricant laxatives, see AGORAL Marshmallow and AGORAL

Plain, respectively, in this section. Dosage for children: 2 ml.

SAFE-TIP OIL RETENTION ENEMA (OTC). Light mineral oil (lubricant laxative). For a profile of lubricant laxatives, see AGORAL Plain in this section. Dosage for children over 2 years of age: 60 ml. a day.

SENAKOT (OTC). Tablets, granules, suppositories. Senna concentrate (stimulant laxative). For a profile of stimulant laxatives, see AGORAL Marshmallow in this section. For children over 60 lb. of body weight, 1 tablet at bedtime, up to 2 tablets 2 times a day; ½ teaspoon of granules at bedtime, up to 1 teaspoon 2 times a day; ½ suppository at bedtime.

SENAKOT-S Tablets (OTC). Ingredients same as for SENAKOT in this section, plus dioctyl sodium sulfosuccinate (docusate sodium) (lubricant laxative). For a profile of lubricant laxatives, see AGORAL Plain in this section. Dosage for children over 60 pounds of body weight, 1 tablet at bedtime.

SENAKOT Syrup (OTC). Ingredients same as for SENAKOT, in this section, plus alcohol (sedative and solvent). Dosage for children 5 to 15 years of age, 1 teaspoon to 2 teaspoons at bedtime, up to 2 teaspoons 2 times a day; for children 1 year to 5 years of age, ½ to 1 teaspoon at bedtime, up to 1 teaspoon 2 times a day; for children 1 month to 1 year of age, ¼ to ½ teaspoon at bedtime, up to ½ teaspoon 2 times a day.

SURFAK (OTC). Capsules. Dioctyl calcium sulfosuccinate (docusate calcium) (lubricant laxative). For a profile of lubricant laxatives, see AGORAL Plain in this section. Dosage for children over 6 years of age, 50 to 150 mg. a day.

DRUGS TO TREAT DIARRHEA

Trade names
    See list of drugs in this section, page 141.

Ingredients
    See under *How these drugs work* and under individual drugs in this section.

These drugs are used to
    Relieve nonspecific diarrhea—frequent passage of loose stools which has no specific cause.

How these drugs work
    This is how the classes of drugs in antidiarrhea medicine act:
    Binding agents—act to absorb and detoxify. Examples: kaolin and pectin.
    Belladonna alkaloids—act to control spasmodic activity, excess motion, and excessive secretions in the gastrointestinal tract. Example: Hyoscine.
    Opium preparations—act to relieve diarrhea and pain associated with it. Example: paregoric.
    Other chemicals—see under individual drugs in this section.

The FDA has
> ☑ Approved these drugs.*
> ☐ Not approved these drugs.

The drugs

√ *DONNAGEL* (OTC). Elixir, kaolin, pectin (binding agents), hyoscine sulfate, atropine sulfate, and hyoscine hydrobromide (belladonna alkaloids). Do not use these binding agents without your doctor's approval if your child has asthma or stomach ulcer or if your child is taking any other medicine. Side effect of these binding agents is constipation. Do not use belladonna alkaloids if your child has glaucoma or organic pyloric stenosis, and do not use without your doctor's approval if your child has urinary retention. Belladonna drugs should not be used frequently or over extended periods of time and should be discontinued at once if eye pain occurs. Common side effects of belladonna alkaloids are drowsiness, dry mouth, urine retention, fear of light, blurred vision, rapid pulse, and dizziness. Dosage for children over 6 years of age, for children 30 lb. of body weight or more, 1 teaspoon to 2 teaspoons after each bowel movement; for children 20 lb. of body weight, 1 teaspoon; for children 10 lb. of body weight, ½ teaspoon; all doses for children under 6 years of age, every 3 hours, up to 4 doses in 24 hours. ☑ This drug is not approved by the FDA.

DONNAGEL-PG (OTC). Suspension. For treatment of acute nonspecific diarrhea. Opium (opium preparation), kaolin, pectin (binding agents), hyoscyamine sulfate, atropine sulfate, hyoscine hydrobromide (belladonna alkaloids). Do

*See under individual drugs in this section for exceptions.

not use an opium preparation without the approval of your doctor if your child has a chronic lung disease (asthma, bronchitis, or emphysema, for example); heart, kidney, or liver disease; hypothryoidism; Addison's disease (insufficiency of the adrenal glands); colitis; gall bladder disease; or if your child is taking antihistamines, cold medicines; allergy medicines (including hay fever medicines); barbiturates; prescription pain medicines; narcotics; sleep medicines; tranquilizers; sedatives; medicines to treat depression, including MAO (monoamine oxidase) inhibitors; or anesthetics. Common side effects: sweating, fatigue, flushing, red face, urinary problems, dizziness, faintness, light-headedness, drowsiness. *Warning:* Should signs of drowsiness occur, deter your child from engaging in potentially hazardous activities requiring alertness. Opium preparations may be addictive. For profiles of binding agents and belladonna alkaloids and for dosage, see DONNAGEL in this section. ☑ This drug is not approved by the FDA.

√ *KAOPECTATE* (OTC). Liquid. Kaolin and pectin (binding agents). For a profile of binding agents, see DONNAGEL in this section. Dosage to be given after each bowel movement or as needed: for children over 12 years of age, 4 tablespoons; for children 6 to 12 years of age, 2 to 4 tablespoons; for children 3 to 6 years of age, 1 tablespoon to 2 tablespoons; for children under 3 years of age, consult your physician.

√ *LOMOTIL* (℞). For the adjunctive treatment of diarrhea. Tablets, liquid. Diphenyloxylate (a drug related to meperidine, an opiumlike narcotic), atropine sulfate (belladonna alkaloid). For a profile of opium, see DONNAGEL-PG in this section. For a profile of belladonna alkaloids, see DONNAGEL in this section. Dosage, to be given up to daily limits until diarrhea is controlled: for children 8 to 12 years of age, 4 ml. 5 times a day; for children 5 to 8 years of age, 4 ml. 4 times a day; for children 2 to 5 years of age, 4 ml. 3 times a day; for children under 2 years of age, consult your doctor. Warning: Lomotil can be very toxic in children below age 6.

√ *PAREGORIC* (℞). Camphorated tincture of opium. For a profile of opium, see DONNAGEL-PG in this section. Dosage for children: .25 to .5 ml. per kilogram (about 2.2 lb.) 4 times a day until diarrhea is under control.

PAREPECTOLIN (℞). Paregoric (opium preparation), kaolin, pectin (binding agents). For profiles of opium and binding agents, see DONAGEL-PG and DONNAGEL respectively, in this section. Dosage after each bowel movement, but no more than 4 a day; for children 6 years of age or over, 2 teaspoons; for children 3 to 6 years of age, 1 teaspoon; for children 1 year of age, ½ teaspoon.

√ *PEPTO-BISMOL* (OTC). Liquid, tablets. For the treatment of diarrhea, upset stomach, and nausea. Bismuth subsalicylate (a salicylate related to aspirin). Pepto-Bismol acts to control common diarrhea within 24 hours and soothes irritated stomach with a protective coating. Do not use without your doctor's approval if your child is taking blood thinners (anticoagulants), medicines for diabetes or gout, or if diarrhea is accompanied by high fever or continues for 2 days while on this medicine. For a profile of salicylate, see page 151. Dosage, to be repeated ½ to 1 hour as needed, up to 8 doses a day, liquid, for children 10 to 14 years of age, 4 teaspoons; for children 6 to 10 years of age, 2 teaspoons; for children 3 to 6 years of age, 1 teaspoon; tablets, to be repeated every ½ to 1 hour as needed, up to 8 doses a day, for children 6 to 10 years, 1 tablet; for children 3 to 6 years, ½ tablet.

DRUGS TO TREAT GASTROINTESTINAL DISORDERS

I. SPASMS (INCLUDING COLIC)

Trade names
   See list of drugs in this section, page 145.

Ingredients
   See under *How these drugs work* and under individual drugs in this section.

These drugs are used to
   Relieve, mainly, painful spasms of the gastrointestinal tract associated with a variety of disorders of the stomach and intestines.

How these drugs work
   This is how the classes of drugs in medicines to treat gastrointestinal spasms act.
   Antispasmodics—act to smooth muscle spasms. Example: dicyclomine hydrochloride.
   Sedatives—act to calm the nervous system. Example: phenobarbital.

The FDA has
   ☑ Approved these drugs.*
   ☐ Not approved these drugs.

*See under individual drugs in this section for exceptions.

The drugs

√ *BENTYL* (℞). Capsules and syrup. Dicyclomine hydrochloride (antispasmodic). Do not use this drug if your child is sensitive to it, or has certain gastrointestinal, kidney, liver, heart, thyroid, muscular, or eye disorders (consult your doctor), or is receiving medicines for sleep, ulcers, certain nervous disorders, diarrhea, depression, or is taking antacids, antihistamines, amantadine, haloperidol, or MAO (monoamine oxidase) inhibitors. Dosage for children, 1 teaspoon 3 or 4 times a day. Common side effects: constipation, bloated feeling, nausea, vomiting, nervousness, drowsiness. *Warning:* Should signs of drowsiness occur, deter your child from engaging in potentially dangerous activities requiring alertness. ☑ Not approved by the FDA.

BENTYL WITH PHENOBARBITAL (℞). Capsules, syrup. For profiles of Bentyl and phenobarbital (sedative), see BENTYL in this section and page 227, respectively. Dosage for children, 1 capsule or 1 teaspoon 3 or 4 times a day; for infants, ½ teaspoon 3 or 4 times a day.

√ *COMBID* (℞). Capsules. Prochlorperazine (sedative of the phenazine class), isopromanide iodide (antispasmodic). For a profile of phenothiazines and antispasmodics, see page 54 and BENTYL in this section, respectively. For children over 12 years of age, 1 capsule twice a day.

√ *DONNATEL ELIXIR* (℞). Phenobarbital (sedative), hyoscymine sulfate, atropine sulfate, hyoscine hydrobromide (belladonna alkaloids—antispasmodics), and alcohol (sedative and solvent). For profiles of phenobarbital and belladonna alkaloids, see pages 227 and 140, respectively. Dosage for children, administered every 4 to 6 hours, 75 to 80 lb. of body weight, 1 to 1½ teaspoons; 50 lb. of body weight, ¾ to 1 teaspoon; 30 lb. of body weight, ½ teaspoon; 20 lb. of

145

body weight, 1.25 to 2.0 ml.; 10 lb. of body weight, .75 ml. ☑ Not approved by the FDA. Classified by the FDA as ☑ possibly effective for treatment of irritable bowel syndrome.

KINESED (℞). Tablets. Belladonna alkaloids and phenobarbital. For profiles of belladonna alkaloids and phenobarbital, see pages 140 and 227, respectively. Dosage for children 2 to 12 years of age, ½ to 1 tablet, chewed or swallowed whole with liquid.

√ *LIBRAX* (℞). See page 40. Dosage: Consult your doctor.

√ *PEPTO-BISMOL* (OTC). See page 143.

II. HEARTBURN

Trade names
See list of drugs in this section, page 149.

Ingredients
Aluminum hydroxide, magnesium hydroxide. For other ingredients, see under individual drugs in this section. Sodium appears in some heartburn medicines. Consult with your doctor about sodium content if your child has high blood pressure or is on a low-sodium diet.

These drugs are used to
Relieve heartburn—the burning sensation caused by a backflow of stomach acid into the region of the food pipe (esophagus) near the heart. Heartburn is a gastrointestinal, not a heart, disorder.

How these drugs work
By neutralizing the effects of the stomach acids. The drugs that do this are called antacids.

The FDA has
☑ Not disapproved of these drugs.*
☐ Disapproved these drugs.

*The drugs in this section are OTC.

These drugs are
☑ Effective.
☐ Probably effective.
☐ Ineffective.

These drugs should not be used under the following conditions
Sensitivity to any ingredient. Consult your doctor.

Your doctor may not approve use of these drugs under the following conditions
If your child has certain gastrointestinal disorders, the laxative habit, appendicitis or possible appendicitis, or undiagnosed rectal bleeding.

Use of the following drugs decreases the effectiveness of these drugs
None reported.

How these drugs interact with other drugs
Adverse effects may be expected when these drugs are taken at the same time as blood thinners (anticoagulants), heart medicines, laxatives, isoniazid, tetracycline, or nerve medicines.

How these drugs are supplied
See under individual drugs in this section.

Dosage
See under individual drugs in this section. *Caution:* Do not overuse. Should you do so, your child may experience irregular heartbeat, fatigue, confusion, light-headedness, dizziness, or a laxative effect.

Common side effects
Diarrhea, cramps, thirst, nausea.

Effect of long-term use
The use of antacids should be limited to 2 weeks. If your child's symptoms continue after that time, consult your doctor.

After-use effects
None reported.

The drugs

ALKA-SELTZER Effervescent Antacid (OTC). In water, contains mainly sodium citrate and potassium citrate (antacids). Dosage for children, 4 tablets in 24 hours; do not use maximum dosage for more than 2 weeks. The manufacturer reports no precautions or adverse drug reactions or side effects with this dosage.

ALKA-SELTZER Effervescent Pain Reliever and Antacid (OTC). See page 154.

CREAMALIN (OTC). Chewable tablets. Aluminum hydroxide, magnesium hydroxide, sodium. For children over 6 years of age, 2 to 4 tablets as needed, up to 16 tablets a day.

MILK OF MAGNESIA (OTC). Tablets, liquid. Magnesium hydroxide. Dosage: tablets, for children 7 to 14 years of age, 1 tablet 1 to 4 times a day; liquid, for children 1 year to 12 years of age, ½ teaspoon to 1½ teaspoons 1 time to 4 times a day.

WIN GEL (OTC). Tablets, liquid. Aluminum hydroxide, magnesium hydroxide, sodium. Dosage: tablets, for children 6 to 12 years of age, 1 tablet to 2 tablets 4 times daily, up to 8 tablets in 24 hours; liquid, for children 6 to 12 years of age, 1 teaspoon to 2 teaspoons 4 times daily, up to 8 teaspoons in 24 hours.

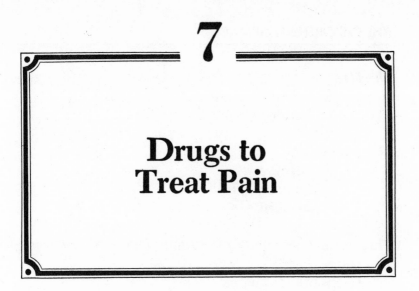

7

Drugs to Treat Pain

I. SALICYLATES

Trade names
   See list of drugs in this section, page 154.

Ingredients
   Acetylsalicylic acid (aspirin) and derivatives. Buffered products help control acidity.

These drugs are used to
   Relieve mild pain (analgesic action), reduce fever (antipyretic action), and reduce swelling and redness (anti-inflammation action).

How these drugs work
   By elevating the pain threshold, acting on the heat-regulating mechanism of the body, and blocking inflammation impulses.

The FDA
☑ Has not disapproved these drugs.*
☐ Has disapproved these drugs.

These drugs are
☑ Effective.
☐ Probably effective.
☐ Ineffective.

These drugs are not to be used under the following conditions
- Sensitivity to salicylates.
- Sensitivity to nonsteroidal anti-inflammatory agents.
- Hemophilia and other bleeding conditions. (Only acetylsalicylates inhibit the formation of blood platelets; consult your doctor about the use of nonacetylsalicylates if your child has a bleeding disorder.)

Your doctor may not approve use of these drugs under the following conditions
- Gastric disorders
- Blood coagulating disorders, and use prior to surgery. (See HEMOPHILIA, above.)
- Asthma, hay fever, nasal polyps (they contribute to sensitivity to these drugs).
- If your child is on a low-sodium diet (for preparations containing high amounts of sodium, see under individual drugs in this section).

Use of the following drug decreases the effectiveness of these drugs
Spironolactone (diuretic).

*Most salacylate analgesics are OTC drugs. The federal government has announced plans to advise parents and doctors against using aspirin to treat children's chicken pox or flulike symptoms because studies have linked this drug to Reye's syndrome, a rare but often fatal children's disease.

152

How these drugs interact with other drugs
- Increase risk of ulceration with corticosteroids, phenylbutazone, oxyphenbutazone, alcohol.
- Increase risk of bleeding with blood thinners (anticoagulants).
- Increase risk of toxicity with methotrexate.
- Produce adverse reactions with medicines for inflammation, nausea, vomiting, arthritis, diabetes, or acidifying or alkalyzing urine; and with vitamin C and antacids.

How these drugs are supplied
See under individual drugs in this section.

Dosage
See under individual drugs in this section. Children are particularly susceptible to overdose. Common overdose symptoms are: diarrhea, severe headache that won't go away, stomach pain, nausea, vomiting, thirst, rapid breathing, sweating, ringing in ears, vision disorders, confusion, dizziness. In young children, overdose can be fatal. Never give your child more than the label recommends. To decrease possible stomach irritation, take with 8 ounces (a glass) of water or milk.

Common side effects
Nausea, vomiting, stomach pain, breathing difficulties, itching, skin rash, loss of hearing, black or tarry stools, gastric bleeding.

Effect of long-term use
Five days in a row is the limit for use of these drugs in children up to 12 years of age. Consult your doctor concerning prolonged use.

After-use effects
   None reported.

The drugs

ALKA-SELTZER Effervescent Pain Reliever and Antacid
(OTC). Tablets. In water, main ingredients are sodium acetylsalicylate and sodium citrate, an antacid. Dosage, 24-
hour period, for children 6 to 12 years of age, 4 tablets; for
children 3 to 5 years of age, 2 tablets; do not use maximum
dosage for more than 5 days. The manufacturer reports no
precautions or adverse drug reactions or side effects with
this dosage.

√ *ANACIN* (OTC). Tablets, capsules. Aspirin (acetylsalicylic
acid), caffeine. Caffeine is a stimulant. Dosage for children
6 to 12, 1 tablet or capsule with water every 4 hours as
needed, up to 10 tablets or capsules per day.

ANACIN MAXIMUM STRENGTH (OTC). See ANACIN in this
section. Dosage for children over 12: Consult your doctor.

ASPERGUM (OTC). Gum tablets to be chewed. For children (or adults) who cannot swallow tablets or gargle
properly. Aspirin (acetylsalicylic acid). For children 6 to 12
years of age, 8 tablets maximum in 24 hours; in children 3
to 6 years of age, 3 tablets maximum in 24 hours.

BAYER ASPIRIN (OTC). Tablets. Aspirin (acetylsalicylic
acid). Dosage for children over 12 years of age, 1 tablet or 2
tablets with water, repeated every 4 hours as necessary, up
to 12 tablets a day; for children under 12 years of age, the
following dosages may be repeated every 4 hours, up to 5
time a day: for children, 11 to under 12 years of age, 1½
tablets; for children 9 to under 11 years of age, 1¼ tablets;
for children 6 to under 9 years of age, 1 tablet; for children

4 to under 6 years of age, ¾ tablet; for children under 2 years of age, consult your doctor.

✓ *BAYER CHILDREN'S CHEWABLE ASPIRIN* (OTC). Orange-flavored tablets. Chewable tablets can be chewed, or crushed, or dissolved in liquid, or swallowed whole. Aspirin (acetylsalicylic acid). Dosage for children may be repeated every 4 hours, but not more than 5 times a day; for children 12 years of age or over (84 lb. of body weight or over), 8 tablets; for children 11 to 12 years of age (77 to 83 lb. of body weight), 6 tablets; for children 9 to 11 years of age (66 to 76 lb. of body weight), 5 tablets; for children 6 to 9 years of age (46 to 65 lb. of body weight), 4 tablets; for children 4 to 6 years of age (36 to 45 lb. of body weight), 3 tablets; for children 2 to 4 years of age (27 to 35 lb. of body weight), 2 tablets; for children under 2 years of age, consult your doctor.

BAYER TIME-RELEASED ASPIRIN (OTC). Tablets. For long-range lasting release. Aspirin (acetylsalicylic acid). Dosage for children over 12 years of age, 1 tablet every 8 hours; for children under 12 years of age, consult your physician.

BUFFERIN (OTC). Tablets. Aspirin (acetylsalicylic acid), buffered. Dosage for children 6 to 12 years of age, 1 tablet every 4 hours, up to 6 tablets in 24 hours; for children under 6 years of age, consult your doctor.

EMPIRIN Analgesic Tablets (OTC). Aspirin (acetylsalicylate). Dosage for children: see under BAYER ASPIRIN in this section.

EXCEDRIN (OTC). Aspirin (acetylsalicylate), acetaminophen (analgesic), salicylamide (salicylate), caffeine (stimulant). For a profile of acetaminophen, see page 157. For children 6 to 12, 1 tablet every 4 hours as needed, up to 4 tablets in 24 hours.

EXTRA-STRENGTH BUFFERIN (OTC). See BUFFERIN in this section. Dosage for children over 12, consult your doctor.

√ *ST. JOSEPH ASPIRIN FOR CHILDREN* (OTC). Chewable orange-flavored tablets. Aspirin (acetylsalicylic acid). Dosage, see under ST. JOSEPH ASPIRIN FOR CHILDREN, page 94.

II. ACETAMINOPHEN

Trade names
   See list of drugs in this section, page 159.

Ingredient
   Acetaminophen.

These drugs are used to
   Reduce mild pain (analgesic action) and fever (antipyretic action). Unlike aspirin, acetaminophen has no anti-inflammation action.

How these drugs work
   By elevating the pain threshold and acting on the heat-regulating mechanism of the body.

The FDA
   ☑ Has not disapproved these drugs.*
   ☐ Has disapproved these drugs.

These drugs are
   ☑ Effective.
   ☐ Probably effective.
   ☐ Ineffective.

*Most acetaminophen analgesics are OTC.

These drugs are not to be used under the following condition
- Sensitivity to this drug.

Your doctor may not approve use of these drugs under the following conditions
- Severe kidney disease.
- Liver disease.
- If your child is sensitive to acetaminophen.
- If your child's symptoms do not improve or if they worsen.
- If fever persists longer than 3 days or resumes after it has subsided.

Use of the following drugs decreases the effectiveness of these drugs
None reported.

How these drugs interact with other drugs
- May interfere with the action of Wafarin, a blood thinner (anticoagulant).

How these drugs are supplied
See under individual drugs in this section.

Dosage
See under individual drugs in this section. Do not exceed recommended dosage; signs of overdose, which can be extremely dangerous in young children, are diarrhea, nausea, vomiting, stomach cramps or stomach pains. Giving your child other medicines containing acetaminophen can lead to overdose (read labels; consult your doctor).

Common side effects

None, but some children may experience fatigue, sore throat, fever, yellowing of eyes or skin, itching, skin rash, bleeding, or bruising.

Effect of long-term use

Do not give to your child for more than 5 consecutive days to avoid possible undesirable effects.

After-use effects

None reported.

The drugs

DATRIL (OTC). Tablets. Acetaminophen. Dosage for children 6 to 12 years of age, 1 tablet every 1 to 4 hours as needed.

DATRIL™ 500 (OTC). See DATRIL, above. Dosage for children over 12 years of age: Consult your doctor.

EXCEDRIN (OTC). Tablets, capsules. Acetaminophen, aspirin (acetylsalicylic acid). For a profile of aspirin, see page 151. For children 12 and over, 1 tablet or capsule every 4 hours as needed.

TYLENOL (CHILDREN'S TYLENOL) (OTC). Chewable tablets. Fruit-flavored. Acetaminophen. Dosage: Doses may be repeated 4 to 5 times a day, up to 5 doses in 24 hours; for children 11 to 12 years of age, 6 tablets; for children 9 to 10 years of age, 5 tablets; for children 6 to 8 years of age, 4 tablets; for children 4 to 5 years of age, 3 tablets; for children 2 to 3 years of age, 2 tablets; for children 1 year to 2 years of age, 1½ tablets.

√ *TYLENOL DROPS* (INFANTS' TYLENOL DROPS) (OTC). Fruit-flavored. Acetaminophen, alcohol. Dosage: Doses may be repeated 4 to 5 times a day, up to 5 doses in 24 hours. For children 4 to 5 years of age, 2.4 ml.; for children 2 to 3 years of age, 1.6 ml.; for children 12 to 23 months of age, .8 ml.; for children 4 to 11 months of age, .6 ml.; for children from birth to 3 months of age, .4 ml.

√ *TYLENOL ELIXIR* (CHILDREN'S TYLENOL ELIXIR) (OTC). Cherry-flavored. Acetaminophen, alcohol. Dosage: Doses may be repeated 4 to 5 times a day, up to 5 doses in 24 hours; for children 11 to 12 years of age, 3 teaspoons; for children 9 to 10 years of age, 2½ teaspoons; for children 6 to 8 years of age, 2 teaspoons; for children 4 to 5 years of age, 1½ teaspoons; for children 2 to 3 years of age, ¾ teaspoon; for children 4 to 11 months of age, ½ teaspoon.

III. DRUGS TO TREAT
MODERATE TO SEVERE PAIN

√ *CODEINE* (℞). Tablets, liquid, injectable. For a profile of codeine, see page 79. Dosage, .5 mg. per kilogram (about 2.2 lb.) of body weight 4 to 6 times a day.

√ *DEMEROL* (℞). Tablets, syrup (banana-flavored). Meperidine hydrochloride, an opiumlike narcotic. For a profile of opium, see DONNAGEL-PG, page 141. Dosage, .5 to .8 mg. per kilogram (about 2.2 lb.) of body weight.

√ *TALWIN* (℞). Tablets. Pentazocine hydrochloride. Behaves like an opium-type drug. For a profile of opium, see DONNAGEL-PG, page 141. For children over 12 years of age, 1 tablet every 3 to 4 hours, up to 12 tablets a day; dosage may be doubled at discretion of your doctor.

8

Drugs to Treat Bacterial Infections (Antibiotics and Anti-Infectives)

I. AMINOGLYCOSIDES

Trade names
   See under individual drugs in this section.

Ingredients
   The family of aminoglycosides includes amikacin, gentamicin, kanamycin, neomycin, streptomycin, and tobramycin.

These drugs are used to
   Help overcome body infections due to bacteria.

How these drugs work
   They kill mainly susceptible Gram-negative bacteria. There are two general classes of bacteria, Gram-negative and Gram-positive. Gram-negative bacteria turn pink when treated with Gram stains. Gram-positive bacteria turn purplish-black. Gram-negative bacteria cause infections of

the respiratory tract, bones, and joints, central nervous system (CNS), skin and soft tissues, and abdomen; they also are present in infections from burns and operations; and they are responsible for bacteremia, septicemia, meningitis, brucellosis, granuloma inguinale, chancroid, urinary-tract infections, and infections of the newborn (neonatal sepsis).

The FDA
    ☑ Has approved these drugs.
    ☐ Has not approved these drugs.

These drugs are
    ☑ Effective.
    ☐ Probably effective.
    ☐ Ineffective.

These drugs should not be used under the following condition
- Sensitivity to aminoglycosides.

Your doctor may not approve use of these drugs under the following conditions
    If your child has:
- Kidney disease.
- Myasthenia gravis (see page 39).
- Parkinson's disease (a nervous disease characterized particularly by trembling).
- A disease characterized by loss of hearing and/or balance (eighth-cranial-nerve disease).

Use of the following drugs decreases the effectiveness of these drugs
    None reported.

How these drugs interact with other drugs
- Adverse reactions can be expected when these drugs are used with other aminoglycosides and with some other antibiotics (consult your doctor).

How these drugs are supplied
Mainly as injectables.

Dosage
See under individual drugs in this section.

Common side effects
Nausea, vomiting, thirst, loss of appetite, urinary difficulties (blood may appear in the urine), dizziness, clumsiness, ear disturbances (buzzing, ringing, feeling of fullness, loss of hearing). See STREPTOMYCIN SULFATE in this section for additional side effects for this drug.

Effect of long-term use
May result in growth of microorganisms not affected by these drugs. This is known as superinfection.

After-use effect
None reported.

The drugs

AMIKEN (℞). Amikacin sulfate. Dosage for children, intravenously or intramuscularly, 7.5 mg. per kilogram (about 2.2 lb.) of body weight every 12 hours, or 5 mg. per kilogram every 8 hours; for newborn, intravenously or intramuscularly, initially 10 mg. per kilogram of body weight, then 7.5 mg. per kilogram every 12 hours.

GARAMYCIN (℞). Gentamycin sulfate. Dosage for children, intravenously or intramuscularly, 2 to 2.5 mg. per kilogram (about 2.2 lb.) of body weight every 8 hours; for infants over 1 week of age, 2.5 mg. per kilogram of body weight every 8 hours; for premature infants and newborns 1 week of age or less, 2.5 mg. per kilogram of body weight every 12 hours.

KANTREX (℞). Kanamycin sulfate. Dosage for children, 7.5 mg. per kilogram (about 2.2 lb.) of body weight, intramuscularly, every 12 hours; or up to 15 mg. a day in 2 to 3 equal doses, intramuscularly or intravenously. Consult your doctor for dosage under special conditions.

NEBCIN (℞). Tobramycin. Dosage for children, intravenously or intramuscularly (except newborn), 3 mg. per kilogram (about 2.2 lb.) of body weight, every 8 hours in equally divided doses; consult your doctor about dosage in life-threatening infections; for newborns, 1 week of age or less, up to 4 mg. per kilogram of body weight per day, every 12 hours in equal doses.

STREPTOMYCIN SULFATE (℞). Streptomycin sulfate. Dosage for children, 20 to 40 mg. per day intravenously every 6 to 12 hours (plus other anti-infective preparations). Streptomycin Sulfate is also used to treat diseases other than those listed under *These drugs are used to* in this section; consult your doctor. In addition to side effects common to aminoglycosides, rash, itching, redness, burning sensation in face or mouth, and swelling are possible with the use of Streptomycin Sulfate.

II. CEPHALOSPORINS

Trade names
     See under individual drugs in this section.

Ingredients
     The family of cephalosporins includes cefaclor, cefa-zolin, cephaloridine, cephalothin, and cephradine.

These drugs are used to
     Help overcome body infections due to bacteria and are used mainly to treat infections of the respiratory, urinary, and biliary tracts, and skin, soft-tissue, bone, joint, middle-ear, and genital infections. Some of these drugs are also used to prevent postoperative infection.

How these drugs work
     They kill susceptible bacteria.

The FDA has
          ☑ Approved these drugs.
          ☐ Not approved these drugs.

These drugs
          ☑ Are effective.
          ☐ Are probably effective.
          ☐ Are not effective.

These drugs should not be used under the following condition
- Sensitivity to cephalosporins or penicillins.

Your doctor may not approve use of these drugs under the following condition
- If your child has kidney disease.

Use of the following drugs decreases the effectiveness of these drugs
None reported.

How these drugs interact with other drugs
- Probenecid may increase toxicity of cephalosporins.
- Adverse reactions may occur when other antibiotics are used; consult your doctor.

How these drugs are supplied
See under individual drugs in this section.

Dosage
See under individual drugs in this section.

Common side effects
Nausea, vomiting, stomach pain and cramps, diarrhea, rash, itching, redness, soreness of mouth and tongue, swelling.

Effect of long-term use
May result in growth of microorganisms not affected by these drugs. This is known as superinfection.

After-use effects
No adverse effects reported.

The drugs

ANCEF (℞). Vials. Cefazolin sodium. Dosage, for mild to moderately severe infections: children 1 month of age or over, 25 to 50 mg. per kilogram (about 2.2 lb.) of body weight 3 to 4 times a day in equal doses; for severe infections, up to 100 mg. per day 3 or 4 times a day in equal doses.

ANSPOR (℞). Capsules, suspension. Cephradine. Dosage for respiratory, skin, and soft-tissue infections: for children 9 months of age or over, 25 to 50 mg. per kilogram (about 2.2 lb.) of body weight a day, every 6 or 12 hours in divided doses; in severe or chronic cases, dosage may be increased to 1 gm. (1,000 mg.)

√ *CECLOR* (℞). Capsules, suspension. Cefaclor. Dosage for children 1 month of age or over, 20 mg. per kilogram (about 2.2 lb.) of body weight a day every 8 hours in divided doses; for more serious infections, from 40 mg. per kilogram to 1 gm. (1,000 mg.) per day (consult your doctor).

CEFADYL (℞). Vials. Cephaparin sodium. Dosage for children 3 months of age or over, 40 to 80 mg. per kilogram (about 2.2 lb.) of body weight per day, intravenously or intramuscularly, in equal doses.

√ *KEFLEX* (℞). Suspension, pediatric drops. Cephalexin. Dosage for children, 25 to 50 mg. per kilogram (about 2.2 lb.) of body weight per day in 4 divided doses; double dosage for severe infections; 75 to 100 mg. per kilogram per day for otitis media (an infection of the middle ear).

KEFLIN (℞). Vials. Cephalothin sodium. Dosage for children, 80 to 160 mg. per kilogram (about 2.2 lb.) of body weight, intramuscularly or intravenously, in divided doses.

KEFZOL (℞). See ANCEF in this section.

MANDOL (℞). Vials. Cefamandole nafate. For children 6 months of age or over, 100 mg. per kilogram (about 2.2 lb.) of body weight a day, intramuscularly or intravenously, in equal doses every 4 to 8 hours; in severe cases, up to 150 mg. per kilogram per day, as in preceding instructions.

MEFOXIN Vials (℞). Cefoxitin sodium. Dosage for children 3 months of age or over, 50 to 160 mg. per kilogram (about 2.2 lb.) of body weight, intramuscularly or intravenously, in 4 equally divided dosages.

VELOSEF (℞). See ANSPOR in this section.

III. PENICILLINS

Trade names
    See under individual drugs in this section.

Ingredients
    The family of penicillins is divided into two types, penicillinase-sensitive and penicillinase-resistant. There are a number of drugs in each type. In this section, penicillinase-sensitive pencillins are designated PS; penicillinase-resistant penicillins, PR.

These drugs are used to
    Help overcome body infections due to bacteria. Some PS penicillins are used to treat infections of the ear, nose, throat, lower respiratory tract (air passage leading to the lungs), genitourinary tract, skin, soft tissue, and infections of newborn infants (neonatal sepsis). Some PR penicillins are used to treat mild to moderate upper respiratory infections, severe lower respiratory infections, and skin, soft tissue, and disseminated infections. For other PS and PR uses, see under individual drugs in this section.

How these drugs work
    They kill susceptible bacteria.

The FDA has
        ☑ Approved these drugs.
        ☐ Not approved these drugs.

These drugs are
    ☑ Effective
    ☐ Probably effective.
    ☐ Not effective.

These drugs should not be used under the following condition
    • Sensitivity to penicillins.

Your doctor may not approve use of these drugs under the following conditions
    If your child has:
    • General allergies (if general allergies are present, the penicillin should be tested for allergy potential before it is administered).
    • Kidney disease (see exceptions under individual drugs in this section).

Use of the following drugs decreases the effectiveness of these drugs
    Tetracyclines. Also see PENICILLIN in this section.

How these drugs interact with other drugs
    • You can expect adverse reactions if your child is taking certain other antibiotics (consult your doctor).

How these drugs are supplied
    See under individual drugs in this section.

Dosage
    See under individual drugs in this section. Give 1 hour prior to meals, or 2 hours after meals, with 8 ounces (1 glass) of water, except for amoxicillins, which may be taken at any time. When used as a liquid, amoxicillin may be mixed with formulas and cold soft drinks and taken immediately after mixing.

Common side effects

Sore mouth or tongue, hives, rash, itching. For other side effects, see under individual drugs in this section. Overdose may result in severe diarrhea, nausea, or vomiting. If severe wheezing begins, emergency measures may be required. Should your child show these symptoms, consult your doctor.

Effect of long-term use

May result in growth of microorganisms not affected by these drugs. This is known as superinfection.

After-use effects

No adverse effects reported.

The drugs

√ *AMCILL* (℞). See POLYCILLIN in this section.

√ *AMOXIL* (℞). Capsules, suspension, pediatric drops. Amoxicillin (PS). Dosage for ear, nose, throat, genitourinary tract, skin, and soft tissue infections: for children under 6 kg. (about 13.2 lb.) of body weight, 25 mg. or .5 ml. every 8 hours; for children 6 to 8 kg. (about 13.2 to 17.6 lb.) of body weight, 50 mg. or 1 ml. every 8 hours; for children less than 20 kg. (about 44 lb.) of body weight, 20 mg. per kilogram (about 2.2 lb.) of body weight every 8 hours in divided doses, which can be doubled in severe cases; for children 20 kg. or more of body weight, 250 mg. every 8 hours, which can be doubled for severe infections. Dosage for lower respiratory tract infections: for children under 6 kg. (about 13.2 lb.) of body weight, 50 mg. or 1 ml. every 8 hours; for children 6 to 8 kg. (about 13.2 to 17.6 lb.) of body weight, 100 mg. or 2 ml. every 8 hours; for children less than 20 kg. (about 44 lb.) of body weight, 40 mg. per kg. (about 2.2 lb.) of body weight in divided doses every 8 hours; for children 20 kg. or more of body weight, 500 mg. every 8 hours. See DOSAGE in this section.

BETAPEN-VK (R). See PEN-VEE K in this section.

√ *BICILLIN L-A* (R). Vials, cartridge needle units, syringe. Penicillin G benzathine (PS). Dosage to treat certain bacterial upper respiratory tract infections: for children under 60 lb. of body weight, 300,000 to 600,000 units, intramuscularly in 1 dose; for children over 60 lb. of body weight, 900,000 units, intramuscularly in a single dose. Dosage to treat congenital syphilis, children 2 to 12 years of age, consult your doctor. Additional side effects are nausea, vomiting, and diarrhea. Effectiveness of penicillin G may be decreased by acidic beverages (orange or grapefruit juice, for example) taken within one hour of dose.

CYCLAPEN-W (R). Tablets, suspension. Cyclacillin (PS). Dosage for treatment of tonsilitis and pharyngitis: for children under 25 kg. (about 45 lb.) of body weight, 125 mg. 4 times daily, spaced equally; for children over 25 kg. of body weight, double the dosage. Dosage for treatment of otitis media (a disease of the middle ear) and skin infections: children, 50 to 100 mg. daily, in 4 doses, equally spaced. Dosage for treatment of mild bronchitis and pneumonia: 50 mg. per kilogram (about 2.2 lb.) of body weight in 4 doses, equally spaced. Dosage for chronic bronchitis, pneumonia, and urinary tract infections, 100 mg. per kilogram (about 2.2 lb.) per day in 4 doses, equally spaced. Additional side effects are nausea, vomiting, and diarrhea.

√ *DYNAPEN* (R). Capsules, suspension. Dicloxacillin sodium (PR). Dosage for severe infections of lower respiratory tract, children less than 40 kg. (about 88 lb.) of body weight, 25 mg. per kilogram (about 2.2 lb.) per day every 6 hours, doses divided equally. Nausea, vomiting, and diarrhea are less common than with PS penicillins.

GEOPEN (℞). Vials. Carbenicillin disodium (PS). Dosage for urinary tract infections: for children, 50 to 200 mg. per kilogram (about 2.2 lb.) a day, intramuscularly or intravenously, 4 to 6 times a day in divided doses. Dosage for certain body, respiratory, soft tissue infections, and meningitis: for children, 400 to 500 mg. per kilogram (about 2.2 lb.) a day by continuous infusion or in divided doses. Dosage for other body, respiratory, and soft tissue infections: for children, 300 to 500 mg. per kilogram (about 2.2 lb.) a day by continuous infusion or in divided doses (consult your doctor). Dosage for infections of the newborn (neonatal sepsis): for children under 2 kg. (about 4.4 lb. of body weight), 100 mg. per kilogram (about 2.2 lb.) of body weight, intramuscularly or intravenously initially, then 75 mg. the same way every 8 hours during first week after birth, then 100 mg. per kilogram of body weight, the same way thereafter; for children over 2 kg. of weight, the same as for children under 2 kg. of weight, except 3 days after birth, increase dose to 100 mg. Additional side effects are nausea, vomiting, and diarrhea.

√ *LAROTID* (℞). See AMOXIL in this section.

√ *OMNIPEN* (℞). See POLYCILLIN in this section.

√ *PENTID* (℞). Tablets, syrup. Penicillin G potassium (PS). Dosage for children under 12 years of age, 15 to 56 mg. per kilogram (about 2.2 lb.) a day in 3 to 6 divided doses. Additional side effects are nausea, vomiting, and diarrhea.

√ *PEN-VEE K* (℞). Tablets, solution. Penicillin V potassium. Dosage, for children before dentistry or minor surgery of upper respiratory tract to prevent bacterial heart infection should your child have heart lesions: under 60 lb. of body weight, 1 gm. ½ to 1 hour before procedures, then 250 mg. every 6 hours, up to 8 doses; for children 60 lb. of body weight or over, double the dosage.

√ *POLYCILLIN* (℞). Capsules, suspension, pediatric drops. Ampicillin (PS). Dosage to treat respiratory tract and soft tissue infections: oral, for children under 20 kg. (about 44 lb.) of body weight, 50 mg. per kilogram (about 2.2 lb.) every 6 to 8 hours in equally divided doses; for children 20 kg. of body weight or more, 250 mg. every 6 hours. Dosage to treat gastronintestinal and urinary tract infections: for children less than 20 kg. (about 44 lb.) of body weight, 100 mg. per kilogram (about 2.2 lb.) of body weight every 6 to 8 hours in equally divided doses; for children 20 kg. or over, 500 mg. every 6 hours. Additional common side effects: nausea, vomiting, and diarrhea.

POLYCILLIN-N (℞). Vials. Ampicillin sodium (PS). Dosage to treat respiratory tract and soft tissue infections: intramuscular or intravenous, for children under 40 kg. (about 88 lb.) of body weight, 25 to 50 mg. every 6 to 8 hours in divided doses; for children 40 kg. of body weight or more, 250 to 500 mg. every 6 hours. Dosage to treat gastronintestinal and urinary tract infections: for children under 40 kg. (about 88 lb.) of body weight, 50 mg. per kilogram (about 2.2 lb.) of body weight per day; for children 40 kg. or more of body weight, 500 mg. every 6 hours; for severe-case dosages, consult your doctor. Additional common side effects: nausea, vomiting, and diarrhea.

√ *POLYMOX* (℞). See AMOXIL in this section.

√ *PRINCIPEN* (℞). See POLYCILLIN-N above.

PRINCIPEN/N (℞). See POLYCILLIN-N in this section.

PROSTAPHLIN (℞). Capsules, solution, vials. Oxacillin sodium (PR). Dosage for mild to moderate upper respiratory, skin, and soft tissue infections: for children, oral, less than 40 kg. (about 88 lb.) of body weight, 50 mg. per kilogram (about 2.2 lb.) per day, doses divided equally; by injection, intramuscularly or intravenously, same as for oral; for children 40 kg. or more of body weight, 500 mg. every 4 to 6 hours for 5 days. Dosage to treat severe lower respiratory tract or severe infections: by injection, intramuscularly or intravenously, children less than 40 kg. (about 88 lb.) of body weight, 100 mg. per kilogram (about 2.2 lb.) of body weight every 4 to 6 hours; orally, 100 mg. per kilogram per day every 4 to 6 hours in equally divided doses. Nausea, vomiting, and diarrhea are not as common side effects as with some PS penicillins.

PYOPEN (℞). Vials. Carbenicillin disodium (PS).

ROBICILLIN-VK (℞). See PEN-VEE K in this section.

√ *SK-AMPICILLIN* (℞). See POLYCILLIN in this section.

√ *SK-PENICILLIN-VK* (℞). See PEN-VEE K in this section.

√ *TEGOPEN* (℞). Capsules, solution. Cloxacillin sodium (PR). Dosage for mild to moderate upper respiratory, skin, and soft tissue infections: for children under 20 kg. (about 44 lb.) body weight, 50 mg. per kilogram (about 2.2 lb.) per day every 6 hours in equally divided doses; for severe lower respiratory tract and disseminated infections, double dosage. Nausea, vomiting, and diarrhea are not as common side effects as with some PS penicillins.

TICAR (℞). Vials. Ticarcillin disodium (PS). Dosage to treat respiratory tract, intra-abdominal, female pelvic and genital tract, skin and soft tissue infections, and bloodstream infections: for children under 40 kg. (about 88 lb.) of body weight, 200 to 300 mg. per kilogram (about 2.2 lb.) of body weight per day, intravenously, every 4 to 6 hours in divided doses; for children 40 kg. of body weight or over, the same dose every 3, 4, or 6 hours. Dosage to treat uncomplicated genitourinary tract infections: for children under 40 kg. (about 88 lb.) of body weight, 50 to 100 mg. per kilogram (about 2.2 lb.) of body weight per day, intravenously or intramuscularly, every 6 to 8 hours in divided doses; for complicated infections, 1 gm. (1,000 mg.) intravenously or intramuscularly every 6 hours, or 150 to 200 mg. per kilogram (about 2.2 lb.) of body weight per day, intravenously, in divided doses. Dosage for infection in newborn children (neonatal sepsis): for children under 2 kg. (about 4.4 lb.) of body weight, 100 mg., intravenously or intramuscularly, as initial dose, then 75 mg. in the same way every 8 hours during first week after birth, followed by 100 mg. per kilogram (about 2.2 lb.) in the same way every 4 hours; for children over 2 kg., dosage is every 4 to 6 hours during first 2 weeks after birth, followed by same dosage as for children under 2 kg. Additional common side effects: nausea, vomiting, diarrhea.

√ *TOTACILLIN* (℞). See POLYCILLIN-N in this section.

TOTACILLIN-N (℞). See POLYCILLIN-N in this section.

√ *TRIMOX* (℞). See AMOXIL in this section.

√ *UTICILLIN VK* (℞). See PEN-VEE K in this section.

√ *V-CILLIN K* (℞). See PEN-VEE K in this section.

√ *VEETIDS* (℞). See PEN-VEE K in this section.

IV. TETRACYCLINES

Trade names
   See under individual drugs in this list.

Ingredients
   Tetracyclines, a family of antibiotic drugs.

These drugs are used to
   Help overcome body infections due to bacteria. These include urinary tract, skin, and soft tissue infections, rickettsia, as well as other infections arising from many types of bacteria.

How these drugs work
   They kill susceptible bacteria.

The FDA has
       ☑ Approved these drugs.
       ☐ Not approved these drugs.

These drugs are
       ☑ Effective.
       ☐ Probably effective.
       ☐ Not effective.

These drugs should not be used under the following conditions
   • Sensitivity to tetracyclines.

- Sensitivity to procaine-type anesthetics (for exceptions, see under individual drugs in this section).

Your doctor may not approve use of these drugs under the following conditions
If your child has:
- Liver disease.
- Kidney disease (for exceptions, see under individual drugs in this section).

Use of the following drugs decreases the effectiveness of these drugs
Antacids, iron supplements, sodium bicarbonate. Do not give your child milk or dairy products, or a formula containing milk within 1 to 2 hours of a tetracycline dose, since these foods decrease the effect of the drug (for exceptions, see under individual drugs in this section).

How these drugs interact with other drugs
Adverse reactions can be expected when these drugs are taken at the same time as calcium supplements, magnesium-containing laxatives, magnesium salicylate, aminosalicylate calcium, or penicillins.

How these drugs are supplied
See under individual drugs in this section.

Dosage
See under individual drugs in this section. No dose is permitted to children under 8 years of age.

Common side effects
Discolored tongue, sore tongue or mouth, nausea, vomiting, diarrhea, stomach cramps, burning sensation in stomach, rectal or genital itching, sensitivity to sunlight.

Effects of long-term use
May result in growth of microorganisms not affected by these drugs. This is known as superinfection.

After-use effects
No adverse side effects reported.

The drugs

ACHROMYCIN (℞). Vials. Tetracycline hydrochloride. Dosage for children over 8 years of age: 25 mg. per kilogram (about 2.2 lb.) of body weight every 8 to 12 hours, intramuscularly, in single or divided doses; or 6 mg. per kilogram of body weight, intravenously, 3 times a day, or up to 10 to 12 mg. per day. Do not use if your child is sensitive to procaine or related drugs.

√ *ACHROMYCIN V* (℞). Capsules, syrup. Tetracycline hydrochloride. Dosage for children over 8 years of age: 25 to 50 mg. per kilogram (about 2.2 lb.) of body weight, in 2 to 4 doses, equally divided.

√ *MINOCIN* (℞). Capsules, syrup, vials. Minocycline hydrochloride. Dosage for children over 8 years of age: oral and by intravenous injection, 4 mg. per kilogram (about 2.2 lb.) of body weight initially, then 2 mg. per kilogram every 12 hours. Your doctor may approve use of this drug if your child has a kidney disease. Your child may take milk products or other food with each dose if this drug produces upset stomach. Sensitivity to sunlight is unusual, but in addition to other tetracycline effects, dizziness, unsteadiness, and light-headedness can be produced by minocycline.

√ *SUMYCIN* (℞). See ACHROMYCIN in this section.

TERRAMYCIN (℞). Tablets, capsules, syrup. Oxytetracycline. Dosage: oral, for children over 8 years of age, 25 to 50 mg. per kilogram (about 2.2 lb.) of body weight per day in 4 doses, divided equally; by injection, 15 to 25 mg. per kilogram per day intramuscularly in 1 dose, or every 8 to 12 hours in equal doses; in severe cases, 6 mg. per kilogram 2 times a day intravenously, up to 10 mg. per kilogram per day.

√ *TETREX* (℞). Capsules. Tetracycline phosphate complex. Dosage: for children over 8 years of age and up to 40 kg. (about 88 lb.) of body weight, 25 mg. per kilogram (about 2.2 lb.) of body weight per day, in 4 doses, divided equally; for children over 8 years of age and over 40 kg. of body weight, 250 mg. 4 times a day, or 500 mg. 2 times a day, equally divided.

VIBRAMYCIN (℞). Capsules, syrup, suspension, vials. Doxycycline. Dosage, oral: for children over 8 years of age and up to 100 lb. of body weight, 2 mg. per pound, in 2 divided doses initially, then 1 mg. (2 mg. in severe cases) per pound of body weight daily in a single dose, or 2 doses equally divided; for children over 8 years of age and over 100 lb., 100 mg. every 12 hours initially, then 100 mg. daily in a single dose, or 2 doses equally divided, or every 12 hours in severe cases. Dosage by injection: 2 mg. per pound intravenously in 1 to 2 infusions initially, then 1 to 2 mg. per pound in 1 to 2 infusions; for children over 8 years of age and over 100 lb., 200 mg. intravenously in 1 to 2 infusions initially, then 100 to 200 mg. per day. Your doctor may not approve use of this drug if your child has kidney disease. Your child may take milk products or other food with each dose if this drug produces upset stomach.

V. ERYTHROMYCINS

Trade names
>See under individual drugs in this section.

Ingredients
>Erythromycins, a family of antibiotic drugs.

These drugs are used to
>Help overcome body infections due to bacteria. These include mild to moderate infections of the respiratory tract, skin, and soft tissue, plus a number of other diseases (consult your doctor). They are often prescribed when your child is sensitive to penicillin.

How these drugs work
>They kill susceptible bacteria.

The FDA has
>☑ Approved these drugs.
>☐ Not approved these drugs.

These drugs are regarded as **particularly** safe antibiotics.

These drugs are
>☑ Effective.
>☐ Probably effective.
>☐ Not effective.

These drugs should not be used under the following condition
> • Sensitivity to erythromycins.

Your doctor may not approve use of these drugs under the following condition
> If your child has:
> • Liver disease.

Use of the following drugs decreases the effectiveness of this drug
> None reported.

How these drugs interact with other drugs
> • Adverse reactions can be expected when these drugs are taken with other antibiotics (consult your doctor).

Dosage
> See under individual drugs in this section. Most erythromycins are taken 1 hour before, or 3 to 4 hours after, meals (for exceptions, see individual drugs in this section).

Common side effects
> Nausea, vomiting, diarrhea, soreness of tongue and mouth, stomach cramps, and stomach disorders. *Caution:* In some children, this drug can cause yellowing of skin and eyes, fatigue, stomach pain, dark or amber-colored urine, pale stools. Should any of these symptoms occur, consult your doctor at once, and do not resume dosage without approval.

Effect of long-term use
> May result in growth of microorganisms not affected by these drugs. This is known as superinfection.

After-use effects
   None reported.

The drugs

√ *BRISTAMYCIN* (℞). See E-MYCIN, below.

√ *E.E.S* (℞). See E-MYCIN, below.

√ *E-MYCIN* (℞). Tablets. Erythromycin. Dosage: for children with mild to moderate infections, 30 to 50 mg. per kilogram (about 2.2 lb.) of body weight per day, divided doses; with severe infections, 60 to 100 mg. per kilogram per day. For dosage for special uses of this drug, consult your doctor.

√ *E-MYCIN E* (℞). Suspension. Erythromycin ethylsuccinate. See E-MYCIN, above. This drug may be taken at meals or on a full stomach.

√ *ERYTHROCIN* (℞). See E-MYCIN, above.

ERYTHROCIN LACTOBIONATE—I.V. Vials (℞). Erythromycin lactobionate. Dosage: for severe infections, 15 to 20 mg. per kilogram (about 2.2 lb.) of body weight per day, intravenously; for extremely severe infections, up to 4 gm. (4,000 mg.) a day. For dosage for special uses of this drug, consult your physician.

√ *ERYTHROCIN STEARATE* (℞). Tablets. Erythromycin stearate. Dosage for children, 30 to 50 mg. per kilogram (about 2.2 lb.) of body weight per day in 3 to 4 doses, spaced evenly. For dosage for special uses of this drug, consult your physician. Some brands of this drug may be taken with meals as well as between meals; consult your doctor.

For some infections, sulfonamides are used in conjunction with this drug.

√ *ETHRIL* (℞). See E-MYCIN in this section.

ILOSONE (℞). Capsules, tablets, chewable tablets, suspensions, drops. Erythromycin estolate. Dosage for children, 30 to 50 mg. per kilogram (about 2.2 lb.) of body weight per day, divided doses; for severe infections, double the dosage. For dosages for special uses of this drug, consult your doctor. See COMMON SIDE EFFECTS in this section for caution regarding side effects which are more common with this drug than with other erythromycins.

√ *PEDIAMYCIN* (℞). See E-MYCIN in this section.

√ *PFIZER-E* (℞). See E-MYCIN in this section.

√ *ROBIMYCIN* (℞). See E-MYCIN in this section.

√ *SK-ERYTHROMYCIN* (℞). See E-MYCIN in this section.

√ *WYAMYCIN* (℞). See E-MYCIN in this section.

VI. SULFONAMIDES

Trade names
　　See under individual drugs in this section.

Ingredients
　　Sulfonamides—"sulfa" drugs—are members of a family of anti-infectives. Sulfonamides are sometimes combined with urinary analgesics and other anti-infectives.

These drugs are used to
　　Treat urinary tract (kidney and bladder) infections and relieve pain and burning sensation often associated with these infections, and to treat otitis media (infection of the middle ear), chronic bronchitis, and other infections.

How these drugs work
　　In susceptible bacteria, sulfonamides block the production of proteins and DNA essential for reproduction. These drugs are known as bacteriostatic anti-infectives. Analgesics relieve pain.

The FDA has
　　　　　　☑ Approved these drugs.
　　　　　　☐ Not approved these drugs.

These drugs are
- ☑ Effective.
- ☐ Probably effective.
- ☐ Ineffective.

These drugs should not be used under the following conditions
- Sensitivity to sulfonamides or other ingredients.
- Certain types of kidney disease.
- Bronchial asthma.

Your doctor may not approve use of these drugs under the following conditions
- If your child has porphyria (a nerve and muscle disease sometimes accompanied by mental disturbances).
- Glucose-6-phosphate dehydrogenase (G6PD) deficiency.

Use of the following drug decreases the effectiveness of these drugs
- Para-aminobenzoic acid (the vitamin PABA).

How these drugs interact with other drugs

Adverse reactions can be expected when these drugs are taken with some antibiotics, oral blood thinners (anticoagulants), oral diabetes drugs, sodium and potassium citrates, and sodium bicarbonate.

How these drugs are supplied

See under individual drugs in this section.

Dosage

See under individual drugs in this section. To be taken

with 8 ounces (a glass) of water 1 hour prior to meals or 2 hours after meals. Consult your doctor about extra amount of water to be given your child daily.

Common side effects
Nausea, vomiting, diarrhea, loss of appetite, headache, dizziness, itching, rash, sensitivity to sunlight. *Caution:* Should your child develop skin rash, sore throat, or yellow skin, do not continue treatment without approval of your doctor.

Effect of long-term use
Bacteria may develop a resistance to the drug.

After-use effects
None reported.

The drugs

AZO GANTRISIN (℞). Tablets. For the treatment of bacterial infections of the urinary tract. Sulfisoxazole (sulfonamide), phenazopyridine hydrochloride (analgesic). For children over 12 years of age, 4 to 6 tablets initially, then 2 tablets 3 times a day for 3 days; when pain is relieved, treatment is continued with sulfisoxazole alone.

√ *BACTRIM PEDIATRIC SUSPENSION* (℞). Cherry-flavored or fruit-licorice-flavored suspension. To treat bacterial infections of urinary tract and otitis media (middle-ear disease). Trimethoprim (anti-infective), sulfamethoxazole (sulfonamide). Dosage for children 10 kilograms (about 22 lb.) of body weight, 1 teaspoon every 12 hours; 20 kilograms (about 44 lb.) of body weight, 2 teaspoons every 12 hours; 30 kilograms (about 88 lb.) of body weight, 4 teaspoons every 12 hours. Bactrim is also supplied in tablets, and in double strength (Bactrim DS); for dosages, consult your doctor.

√ *GANTANOL* (℞). Tablets, suspension. For the treatment of bacterial infections of the urinary tract, otitis media (middle-ear disease), and other infections (consult your doctor). Dosage for children 20 lb. of body weight, .5 gm. or 1 teaspoon initially, then .25 gm. or ½ teaspoon twice a day; for children 40 lb. of body weight, 1 gm. or 2 teaspoons initially, then .5 gm. or 1 teaspoon twice a day; for children 60 lb. of body weight, 1.5 gm. or 3 teaspoons initially, then .75 gm. or 1½ teaspoons twice a day; for children 80 lb. of body weight, 2 gm. or 4 teaspoons initially, then 1 gm. or 2 teaspoons twice a day. Gantanol is also supplied in double-strength tablets (Gantanol DS).

√ *GANTRISIN* (℞). Pediatric suspension, pediatric syrup. For treatment of bacterial infections of the urinary tract, otitis media (middle-ear infection), a type of meningitis, and other infections (consult your doctor). Acetyl sulfisoxazole (sulfonamide). For children 2 months of age or older, 75 mg. per kilogram (about 2.2 lb.) of body weight, then 150 mg. per kilogram 6 times a day in divided doses.

√ *SEPTRA* (℞). Tablets, suspension. For treatment of bacterial infections of the urinary tract, acute otitis media (middle-ear infection), chronic bronchitis, and other infections (consult your doctor). Dosage for urinary tract infections, for children 22 lb. of body weight, ½ tablet or 1 teaspoon every 12 hours for 10 days; for children 44 lb. of body weight, 1 tablet or 2 teaspoons every 12 hours for 10 days; for children 66 lb. of body weight, 1½ tablets or 3 teaspoons every 12 hours for 10 days; for children 88 lb. of body weight, 2 tablets or 4 teaspoons every 12 hours for 10 days. Septra also is supplied in double-strength tablets (Septra DS).

THIOSULFIL (℞). Tablets. Sulfamethizole. For treatment only of bacterial infections of the urinary tract. For children over 2 months of age, 30 to 45 mg. per kilogram (about 2.2 lb.) of body weight per day in 4 doses, divided equally.

9

Drugs to Treat Parasitic and Fungal Infections

DRUGS TO TREAT PARASITIC INFECTIONS

TYPICAL ANTIPARASITICAL DRUG

Trade name
   ANTEPAR (℞).

Ingredient
   Piperazine citrate.

This drug is used to
   Treat pinworm and roundworm infections.

How this drug works
   Paralyzes the parasites so they can be expelled through normal excretion.

The FDA has
    ☑ Approved this drug.
    ☐ Not approved this drug.

This drug is
    ☑ Effective.
    ☐ Probably effective.
    ☐ Ineffective.

This drug should not be used under the following conditions
- Sensitivity to piperazine.
- Liver disorders.
- Kidney disorders.
- Convulsive disorders.

Your doctor may not approve use of this drug under the following conditions
- Severe malnutrition.
- Severe anemia.

Use of the following drug decreases the effectiveness of this drug
    Pyrantel pamoate (see ANTIMINTH in following list of drugs).

How this drug interacts with other drugs
    No significant reactions reported.

How this drug is supplied
    Tablets, syrup.

Dosage
    For roundworm infections, children: 1 dose a day for 2 consecutive days; for children 15 lb. of body weight, 1

tablet or 1 teaspoon; for children 30 lb. of body weight, 2 tablets or 2 teaspoons; for children 45 lb. of body weight, 3 tablets or 3 teaspoons; for children 60 lb. of body weight, 4 tablets or 4 teaspoons; for children 75 lb. of body weight, 5 tablets or 5 teaspoons; for children 90 lb. of body weight, 6 tablets or 6 teaspoons; for children 100 lb. or more of body weight, 7 tablets or teaspoons (maximum daily dose); for pinworm infections, children: 1 dose a day for 7 consecutive days; for children 17 lb. of body weight, 1 tablet or 1 teaspoon; for children 34 lb. of body weight, 2 tablets or 2 teaspoons; for children 51 lb. of body weight, 3 tablets or 3 teaspoons; for children 68 lb. of body weight, 4 tablets or 4 teaspoons; for children 85 lb. of body weight or more, 5 tablets or 5 teaspoons (maximum daily dose).

Common side effects

Nausea, vomiting, stomach cramps and pains, diarrhea, headache, skin rashes, blurred vision, headaches, dizziness, muscular weakness, joint pain, memory defects, and other mental disturbances.

Effect of long-term use

Possible adverse effect on the nervous system. Long-term use should be avoided.

After-use effects

No adverse effects reported.

OTHER ANTIPARASITICAL DRUGS

ANTIMINTH (℞). Suspension. For treatment of pinworm and roundworm infections. Pyrantel pamoate. Dosage for children over 2 years of age, 11 mg. per kilogram (about 2.2 lb.) of body weight in 1 dose (with fruit juice or milk if desired). Piperazine (see ANTEPAR on page 193) decreases efficiency of this drug. Common side effects: nausea, vomiting, cramps, diarrhea, painful and futile effort to discharge urine or feces.

ARALEN HYDROCHLORIDE (℞). Ampules. see ARALEN PHOSPHATE below. Dosage for children, 5 mg. per kilogram (about 2.2 lb.) of body weight, intramuscularly, repeated in 6 hours if needed, up to 10 mg. per kilogram in 24 hours.

ARALEN PHOSPHATE (℞). Tablets. For treatment of acute malarial attacks. (Malaria is caused by protozoa, microscopic parasites.) Chloroquine phosphate. Dosage for children, 10 mg. per kilogram (about 2.2 lb.) of body weight to start, followed by progressively reduced doses at certain time intervals (consult your doctor). Do not use this drug if your child has certain visual problems (consult your doctor). If your child has any of the following disorders, your doctor may not approve use of this drug: liver disease, G6PD disease, psoriasis, porphyria. Common side effects: blurred vision and other eye disorders, reduced hearing and other ear disorders, nausea, vomiting, diarrhea, ab-

dominal cramps, itching and other skin disorders, headache, psychological disorders. Irreversible eye damage,
muscular weakness, and blood disorders may occur with
long-term use.

EMETINE HYDROCHLORIDE (℞). Ampules. Emetine
hydrochloride. For treatment of amebic dysentery and
hepatitis as well as other parasitic infections (consult your
doctor). Dosage, for children under 8 years of age, up to 10
mg. per day; children 8 years of age or over, up to 20 mg.
per day.

√ *EURAX* (℞). Cream and lotion. Crotamiton. For treatment
of scabies, a skin disease caused by the itch mite. Do not
use if your child has inflamed skin or is sensitive to this
product. Dosage: After cleaning entire body, massage with
cream or lotion from chin down; repeat in 24 hours; take
cleansing bath 48 hours after final application, or cleanse
after recommended time based on child's age.

FLAGYL (℞). Tablets. For treatment of acute intestinal
amebiasis and amebic liver abscess (caused by amebas,
microscopic parasites). Metronidazole. Dosage for children, 35 to 50 mg. per kilogram (about 2.2 lb.) of body
weight per 24 hours in 3 divided doses for 10 days. Do not
use this drug if your child is sensitive to it, has or has had
blood disorders, or has an active disease of the central
nervous system. Your doctor may not approve use of this
drug if your child is taking an oral blood thinner (anticoagulant). Common side effects: nausea, vomiting, diarrhea,
loss of appetite, stomach pains, and cramps. Many less
common side effects are associated with the use of this
drug; consult your doctor.

√ *KWELL* (℞). Cream, lotion, shampoo. For treatment of
scabies (itch mite) and head louse and crab louse infec-

tions. Lindane. *Caution:* Use with care in children who are particularly susceptible to the toxic effects of this drug. (Lindane is absorbed through the skin.) Dosage: A single treatment, preferably of shampoo, is usually sufficient. Consult your physician.

MINTEZOL (R). Tablets, suspension. For treatment of pinworm, roundworm, hookworm, and whipworm infections, and for relief of symptoms of trichinosis. Thiabendazole. Dosage for children: For pinworm infections, 25 mg. per kilogram (about 2.2 lb.) of body weight or 1 ml. per pound of body weight 2 times a day, up to 3 gm. (3,000 mg.) per day, for 2 doses; then in 7 days 2 doses of 25 mg. per kilogram of body weight, up to 3 gm. (3,000 mg.) per day, over 2 consecutive days; for roundworm, hookworm, and whipworm infections, same initial dosage as for pinworm infections, except use 4 doses over 2 consecutive days; for trichinosis infections, same initial dosage as for pinworm infections, except use 2 to 4 doses over 2 consecutive days. Common side effects similar to those for Antepar (see ANTEPAR in this chapter). Additional common side effects: skin irritation, eruptions, itching.

PLAQUENIL (R). Tablets. Hydroxychloroquine sulfate. See ARALEN PHOSPHATE in this section.

√ *POVAN* (R). Tablets, suspension. For treatment of pinworm infections. Pyrvinium pamoate. Dosage for children, 5 mg. per kilogram (about 2.2 lb.) of body weight, or 5 ml. per 10 kg. of body weight, up to 350 mg., in a single dose, which may be repeated in 2 to 3 weeks. Common side effects: sensitivity to light, nausea, cramps, diarrhea, vomiting (especially with suspension). *Caution:* Vomit and stools may be red (this drug is a dye), but the coloring is harmless.

√ *VERMOX* (℞). Chewable tablets. To treat pinworm, roundworm, hookworm, and whipworm infections. Mebendazole. Dosage for treatment of pinworm infections, for children over 2 years of age, 100 mg. in 1 dose; repeat after 3 weeks if necessary; for other worm infections, 100 mg. 2 times a day for 3 consecutive days; repeat after 3 weeks if necessary. Common side effects are abdominal pain, and in case of serious infections, diarrhea.

DRUGS TO TREAT FUNGAL INFECTIONS

TYPICAL ANTIFUNGAL DRUGS

Trade name
√ *LOTRIMIN* (R).

Ingredient
Clotrimazole.

This drug is used to
Treat athlete's foot, ringworm, and other fungal skin infections. A fungus is an organism resembling a plant without chlorphyll; it lives on other organisms, living or dead.

How this drug works
Damages the fungal cell membrane so vital elements leak out, resulting in the destruction of the fungus.

The FDA has
☑ Approved this drug.
☐ Not approved this drug.

This drug is
☑ Effective.*

*If child shows no improvement after 4 weeks, consult your doctor.

☐ Probably effective.
☐ Ineffective

This drug should not be used under the following condition
• Sensitivity to clotrimazole or base.

Your doctor may not approve use of this drug under the following conditions
None reported.

How this drug interacts with other drugs
No adverse interactions reported.

How this drug is supplied
Solution, cream.

Dosage
Gently massage affected and surrounding areas in the morning and just before bedtime. Keep drug away from eyes.

Common side effects
Itching, burning, stinging, peeling, blistering, rash, hives.

Effects of long-term use
No adverse effects reported.

After-use effects
None reported.

OTHER ANTIFUNGAL DRUGS

MONISTAT 7 VAGINAL CREAM (℞). For the treatment of vulvovaginal candidiasis, a fungal infection of the external genitals and vagina, rare in children. Miconazole nitrate. Dosage for children: 1 applicatorful inserted into vagina at bedtime for 7 days. Common side effects: burning sensation, itching, irritation; less common, pelvic cramps, rash, hives, headache.

√ *MYCELEX* (℞). See LOTRIMIN in this chapter.

√ *MYCELEX-6* (℞). See LOTRIMIN in this chapter.

√ *MYCOLOG* (℞). Cream and ointment. For treatment of certain fungal and bacterial skin infections as well as infantile eczema (an inflammatory disease of the skin, characterized by redness, itching, formation of lesions, and a watery discharge). Nystatin (antifungic), meomycin sulfate, granicidin (antibiotics), triamcinolone acetonide (anti-inflammatory, anti-itching agent). Dosage for children: Apply ointment in thin film or rub cream into affected area 3 times a day. Avoid prolonged use, and consult your doctor on length of treatment. Common side effects: burning sensation, itching, dry skin.

√ *TINACTIN* (OTC). Cream, solution, powder, powder aerosol. For treatment of athlete's foot, ringworm, and a fungal scalp infection. Tolnaftate. Dosage for children, spread ½-in. ribbon of cream on infected area and rub gently morning and evening; apply 2 to 3 drops of solution on affected area and massage gently morning and evening; sprinkle powder on infected area as well as in shoes and socks; spray powder aerosol on infected area. Side effects: manufacturer reports none.

√ *VIOFORM-HYDROCORTISONE* (℞). Cream, ointment, lotion. For treatment of athlete's foot and other fungal infections as well as eczema (a skin rash of unknown origin). This drug also decreases inflammation. Idiochlor-hydroxyquin (antifungic, antibiotic), hydrocortisone (anti-inflammatory agent). Dosage for children: Apply to infected area in thin layer 3 or 4 times a day, or as directed by your doctor. Common side effects: burning sensation, itching, rash, irritation, dry skin.

10

Drugs to Treat Ear and Eye Disorders

DRUGS TO TREAT EAR DISORDERS

TYPICAL DRUG TO TREAT EAR DISORDERS

Trade name
  √ *AURALGAN OTIC SOLUTION* (℞).

Ingredients
  Antipyrine, benzocaine, dehydrated glycerine.

This drug is used to
  Treat the symptoms of acute middle ear infections (otitis media) and to remove excess hardened (impacted) earwax (cerumen).

How this drug works
  The actions of antipyrine, benzocaine, and dehydrated glycerine combine to reduce pain, discomfort, inflamma-

tion, congestion, and pressure of otitis media. These ingredients also act to loosen hardened earwax.

The FDA has
> ☑ Approved this drug.
> ☐ Not approved this drug.

This drug is
> ☑ Effective.
> ☐ Probably effective.
> ☐ Ineffective.

This drug should not be used under the following conditions
- Sensitivity to any ingredient or to any local anesthetic.
- Perforated eardrum.
- Ear discharge.

Your doctor may not approve use of this drug under the following conditions
Consult your doctor.

Use of the following drugs decreases the effectiveness of this drug
None reported.

How this drug reacts with other drugs
No adverse reaction reported.

How this drug is supplied
Solution.

Dosage
For treatment of acute otitis media: Using dropper, run solution along wall of canal until it is filled, being care-

ful not to touch ear with dropper. Then insert a cotton pledget moistened with this drug into the ear. Repeat every 1 to 2 hours until symptoms disappear.

For removal of earwax: Instill in canal 3 times a day for 2 to 3 days. Before and after removal of wax, insert a cotton pledget moistened with this drug following installation.

Common side effects
Itching or burning in the ear.

Effects of long-term use
No adverse effects reported.

After-use effects
No adverse effects reports.

OTHER DRUGS TO TREAT EAR DISORDERS

AEROSPORIN OTIC SOLUTION (℞). Eardrops. For the treatment of infections of outer and middle ear. Polymixin B sulfate (antibiotic). Dosage for children, 2 to 3 drops 3 or 4 times a day.

AMERICAIN-OTIC (℞). Eardrops. To treat pain and itching of certain ear diseases. Benzocaine (anesthetic). Do not use if your child is sensitive to this drug. Dosage for children 1 year to 12 years of age: Clean ear with swab saturated with this drug; then instill 4 to 5 drops of warmed solution as directed by your doctor. The manufacturer reports no adverse side effects.

CERUMENEX DROPS (℞). Eardrops. For removal of earwax. Triethanolamine polypeptide oleate condensate (an agent that emulsifies and softens earwax). Do not use if your child is sensitive to this drug (ask your doctor about a patch test to determine whether your child has an allergic reaction to this drug). Your doctor may not approve its use if your child has, or may possibly have, middle ear disease (otitis media) or a perforated eardrum. Dosage for children: Fill ear canal while child's head is tilted at 45-degree angle, insert cotton plug for 15 to 30 minutes, as prescribed by your doctor, then flush ear gently with lukewarm water, using soft rubber syringe. *Caution:* Avoid exposing large skin areas to this drug, and do not leave drops in canal for more than 15 to 30 minutes, as prescribed by your doctor. Common side effects: none reported; rare side effects are skin disorders.

√ *CHLOROMYCETIN OTIC* (℞). Eardrops. For treatment of some bacterial infections of the external ear canal. Chloramphenicol. Do not use if child is sensitive to this drug. Dosage for children, 2 to 3 drops in the ear 2 or 3 times a day. There is the possibility of proliferation of organisms not susceptible to this drug (superinfection). Common side effects: local irritation, itching, burning.

COLY-MYCIN S OTIC (℞). Eardrops. For treatment of some bacterial infections of the outer ear canal. Colistin sulfate, neomycin sulfate (antibiotics), hydrocortisone acetate (corticosteroid), thonzonium bromide (a substance which helps the other ingredients make contact with the tissues). Do not use if your child is sensitive to any ingredient, or has cowpox, chicken pox, or a herpes simplex infection. Your doctor may not approve use of this drug if your child has a perforated eardrum or chronic middle ear disease (otitis media). Dosage for children, 2 to 3 drops instilled in the ear 2 or 3 times a day. Consult your doctor about using a cotton wick saturated with this drug instead of drops. Common side effect: sensitive skin.

√ *CORTISPORIN OTIC* (℞). Eardrops. For treatment of some bacterial infections of the outer ear canal. Polymixin B sulfate, neomycin sulfate (antibiotics), hydrocortisone (corticosteroid). Do not use if your child is sensitive to any of these ingredients, or has cowpox, chicken pox, or a herpes simplex infection. Your doctor may not approve use of this drug if your child has a perforated eardrum or chronic middle ear disease (otitis media). Dosage for children, 3 drops instilled in the ear 3 or 4 times a day. Common side effects: stinging and burning in the middle ear, sensitive skin.

√ *LIDOSPORIN OTIC* (R). Eardrops. For the treatment, especially the relief of pain and itching, of certain diseases of the ear canal. Polymixin B sulfate (antibiotic), lidocaine hydrochloride (anesthetic), propylene glycol (water remover). Do not use if your child is sensitive to any of these ingredients. Dosage for children, 2 to 3 drops in the ear 3 or 4 times a day. Long-term use may not be safe. ☑ Not approved by the FDA. Classified by the FDA as ☑ probably effective.

OTOBIONE OTIC SUSPENSION (R). See CORTISPORIN OTIC in this section. Dosage for children, 3 drops in the ear 3 or 4 times a day; maximum treatment, 10 days.

TYMPAGESIC (R). Eardrops. To treat pain and inflammation of certain ear diseases. Phenylephrine hydrochloride, antipyrine, benzocaine. Do not use if your child is sensitive to any of these ingredients. Dosage for children: Instill into ear canal until full, then add cotton plug; repeat every 4 hours if needed. The manufacturer reports no common side effects.

VŌSOL HC OTIC SOLUTION (R). For treatment of infections of the outer ear canal. Hydrocortisone, acetic acid, citric acid in a propylene glycol base. These ingredients combine to provide antibacterial, antifungal, and water-removing action. Do not use if your child is sensitive to any of these ingredients, or has cowpox, chicken pox, or a perforated eardrum. Dosage for children: Saturate a cotton wick with solution, insert in ear, keep moist for 24 hours by adding drops from time to time; then remove wick and instill 5 drops 3 or 4 times a day.

VŌSOL OTIC SOLUTION (℞). Ingredients same as for VŌSOL HC OTIC SOLUTION, except that this preparation does not contain hydrocortisone or citric acid. ☑ Not approved by the FDA. Classified by the FDA as ☑ probably effective.

DRUGS TO TREAT
EYE DISORDERS

The following drugs are prescribed by some doctors foɪ children's eye infections, but either general guidelines for use by children have not been established, or the manufacturer does not provide recommended children's doses.

√ *CHLOROPTIC-P S.O.P.* (R). Ointment. To treat eye infections caused by certain bacteria and help reduce eye inflammation. Chloramphenicol (antibiotic), prednisolone, alcohol, corticosteroid, chlorbutanol (anesthetic). Do not use if your child is sensitive to any of these ingredients. Dosage for children is determined by your doctor. Common side effects: stinging, burning sensation in the eye, skin disorders. Long-term use may result in growth of unaffected microorganisms (superinfection).

√ *CORTISPORIN OPTHALMIC* (R). Ointment. To treat eye infections caused by certain bacteria and to help reduce eye inflammation. Polymixin B sulfate, bacitracin zinc, neomycin sulfate (antibiotics), hydrocortisone (corticosteroid). Do not use if your child is sensitive to any of these ingredients, or has herpes simplex, cowpox, chicken pox, viral infections of the eye, fungal infections, or certain bacterial infections. Dosage for children is determined by your doctor. Common side effects: increased eye pressure and possible development of glaucoma, particularly in long-term use; growth of unaffected organisms, particularly fungi (superinfection).

√ *ISOPTO-CARPINE* (℞). Eyedrops. To treat glaucoma (increased pressure in the eye damages the retina and optic nerve, possibly leading to blindness). Pilocarpine hydrochloride (a drug to reduce pressure within the eye). Do not use if your child is sensitive to this drug. Your doctor may not approve use of this drug if your child has asthma. Dosage for children is determined by your doctor. Common side effects: blurred vision, altered vision, eye pain.

√ *NEOSPORIN OPHTHALMIC SOLUTION* (℞). Eyedrops. To treat certain bacterial eye infections. Polymixin B sulfate, neomycin sulfate, and gramicidin (antibiotics). Do not use if your child is sensitive to any of these ingredients. Dosage for children is determined by your doctor. Common side effect: skin sensitivity. Long-term effect: possible growth of unaffected microorganisms (superinfection).

√ *SODIUM SULAMYD* (℞). Eyedrops, ointment. To treat certain bacterial eye infections. Sulfacetamide sodium (antibiotic). Do not use if your child is sensitive to this drug or is receiving silver preparations. Dosage for children is determined by your doctor. Common side effects: irritation, transient stinging or burning, possibility of growth of unaffected microorganisms (superinfection).

11

Drugs to Treat Convulsions

Trade name
   √ *DILANTIN* (℞).

Ingredients
   Phenytoin or phenytoin sodium, which are hydantoin-type anticonvulsants.

This drug is used to
   Treat epileptic and other types of convulsive seizures.

How this drug works
   The exact mechanism is not known.

The FDA has
   ☑ Approved this drug.
   ☐ Not approved this drug.

This drug is
   ☑ Effective.
   ☐ Probably effective.
   ☐ Ineffective.

This drug should not be used under the following condition
  • Sensitivity to hydantoins.

Your doctor may not approve use of this drug under the following conditions
  If your child has:
  • Diabetes.
  • High blood sugar.
  • Blood disease.

Use of the following drugs decreases the effectiveness of this drug
  • Tricyclic antidepressants (in high doses).
  • Antipsychotics (in high doses).
  • Folic acid (a vitamin of the B complex).
  • Valproic acid (sometimes).
  • Alcohol.

How this drug interacts with other drugs
  Adverse effects can be expected when your child receives this drug at the same time as barbiturates, blood thinners (anticoagulants), corticosteroids, sulfonamides, tricyclic antidepressants, or other drugs (consult your doctor).

How this drug is supplied
  Pediatric suspension, tablets, capsules, powder.

Dosage
  For children, 5 mg. per kilogram (about 2.2 lb.) of body weight per day in 2 to 3 doses, equally divided, then up to 300 mg. per day in doses determined by your doctor: recommended maintenance dose is 4 to 8 mg. per kilogram of body weight per day.

Common side effects

Uncontrollable eye motions, skin rash, nausea, vomiting, constipation, dizziness, gum disorders, loss of some muscular coordination, light-headedness, drowsiness. *Warning:* Should signs of drowsiness occur, deter your child from engaging in any potentially hazardous activity requiring alertness.

Effects of long-term use

Your doctor will consult with you at regular intervals to adjust dosage if necessary.

After-use effects

Do not stop taking this drug abruptly; your doctor may reduce dosage gradually to avoid possible adverse effects.

Trade names

√ Phenobarbitals such as *ESKABARB, LUMINAL, SK-PHENOBARBITAL,* and *SOLFOTON* (all ℞ drugs).

For a profile of phenobarbitals, see page 227. Dosage to treat convulsions in children, oral, 3 to 6 mg. per kilogram (about 2.2 lb.) of body weight a day; slowly, 3 to 5 mg. intramuscularly or intravenously.

Trade name
TEGRETOL (℞).

Ingredient
Carbamazepine.

This drug is used to
Treat epileptic and other types of seizures. Because of its serious side effects and potential toxicity, it is used only when the child has not been helped by other anticonvulsant drugs.

How this drug works
The exact mechanism is not known.

The FDA has
☑ Approved this drug.
☐ Not approved this drug.

This drug is
☑ Effective.
☐ Probably effective.
☐ Ineffective.

This drug should not be used under the following conditions
• Sensitivity to this drug or any tricyclic compound.
• Damage to blood-forming tissues.

Your doctor may not approve use of this drug under the following conditions
• Heart damage.
• Liver damage.
• Kidney damage.

- A history of adverse changes in the blood due to drugs.
- If your child has received carbamazepine previously without finishing the course of treatment.

Use of the following drugs decreases the effectiveness of this drug
MAO (monomaine oxidase) inhibitors.

How this drug interacts with other drugs
No significant interactions reported with drugs normally prescribed for children, other than MAO inhibitors.

How this drug is supplied
Tablets.

Dosage
For children over 15 years of age, 200 mg. 2 times a day initially, then increase gradually by 200 mg. per day increments up to 1,200 mg. a day if needed, in 3 to 4 divided doses until a minimum amount proves effective; maintenance dose is usually 400 to 800 mg. per day; for children 12 to 15 years of age, the same, up to 1,000 mg. per day if needed; for children 6 to 12 years of age, 100 mg. 2 times a day initially, then increase gradually by 100 mg. per day increments up to 1,000 mg. per day if needed, in 3 to 4 divided doses until a minimum amount proves effective; maintenance dose is same as for older children.

Common side effects
Warning: This drug may damage the blood-forming tissues, which may result in death. Signs of this damage include mouth sores, bleeding, bruising, sore throat, and fever. Should any of these side effects occur, consult your doctor at once.

More common side effects are nausea, vomiting, dizziness, unsteadiness, drowsiness. *Warning:* Should signs of drowsiness occur, deter your child from engaging in any potentially hazardous activity requiring alertness.

Effects of long-term use
The use of this drug must be monitored by your doctor throughout the course of therapy.

After-use effect
Abrupt discontinuation may cause seizures.

12

Drugs to Treat Sleep Disorders

DRUGS TO TREAT INSOMNIA

I. BARBITURATES

Note: There is disagreement among pediatricians on the issue of treating children's sleep disorders with barbiturates. While some doctors recommend them, with close monitoring, for children's insomnia, others feel that there are no pediatric circumstances that warrant the use of these drugs. If barbiturates are suggested for your child, ask your doctor why he or she feels this alternative seems appropriate to the case. (You might explore non drug therapies—like counseling—with your physician as well.) If you are still uncertain about exposing your child to barbiturates, seek a second opinion.

Trade names
   See list of drugs in this section, page 227.

Ingredients
   See under specific drugs, beginning on page 227.

These drugs are used to
   Induce sleep at bedtime. They are also used for day-time sedation to treat emotional disorders, including anxiety, and to control epileptic and other seizures. Consult your doctor about additional uses.

How these drugs work
   There are two basic types of sleep: REM (rapid-eye-movement sleep) and non-REM sleep. Dreams occur during REM sleep. Non-REM is deeper sleep. It is divided into four stages, the third and fourth of which are the deepest. In childhood, sleep patterns include more periods of non-REM sleep than during any other time of life. Barbiturates induce sleep but suppress REM sleep as well as the deepest stages of non-REM sleep. Because, in general, barbiturates depress the central nervous system (CNS), they are known as CNS depressants.

These drugs should not be used under the following conditions
   - Sensitivity to barbiturates.
   - Previous addiction to sedative-hypnotic drugs.
   - Liver disorders.
   - Difficulty in breathing due to respiratory disorder.
   - Acute or chronic pain.
   - Circulatory collapse.
   - Porphyria (See page 42).

Your doctor may not approve use of these drugs under the following conditions
- Asthma.
- Uticaria (hives).
- Angioneurotic edema (swelling caused by fluids in various parts of the body).

Use of the following drugs decreases the effectiveness of these drugs
No drugs with this action reported.

How these drugs interact with other drugs
- Increase the depressant effects of other CNS (central nervous system) depressants, including:
  —cold drugs containing antihistamines.
  —allergy drugs, including hay fever drugs, containing antihistamines.
  —other insomnia drugs.
  —sedatives.
  —tranquilizers.
  —anesthetics (surgical and dental).
  —anticonvulsants (drugs to treat epilepsy and other seizures).
  —prescription pain drugs.
  —narcotics.
  —alcohol.
- Decrease the effectiveness of coumarin anticoagulants (blood thinners) and hydrocortisone (a medicine that, among other uses, provides relief from inflammation).
- Barbiturates interact with other drugs less likely to be prescribed for children. Inform your doctor of all drugs your child is taking. While your child is on barbiturates, do not give the child any other drug,

prescription or nonprescription, without the approval of your doctor. Adolescents on barbiturates should be warned that when alcoholic beverages are consumed, acute intoxication can result.

How these drugs are supplied
As oral pills, in orally taken liquid form, in vials for injection, and as rectal suppositories.

Dosage
See individual drugs, beginning on page 227.

Common side effects
Nausea, vomiting, hangover, dizziness, light-headedness, lethargy, drowsiness, depression, impaired breathing, headache, slurred speech, pains in muscles and joints, diarrhea. *Warning:* Barbiturates taken at bedtime may decrease alertness the following day. Should this side effect occur, keep young children away from potentially harmful toys and machines, deter adolescents from driving, and keep all children from engaging in potentially hazardous activities requiring alertness.

Effect of long-term use
Possibly addictive.

After-use effects
For a time, your child may sleep poorly, dream more frequently, experience nightmares and hallucinations, feel faint and restless, and go into convulsions or have seizures.

The drugs
Barbiturates recommended for children's use by the manufacturers are listed alphabetically by product name. The ingredient of each product is given, as well as dosage

and other pertinent information not covered in the general description.

AMYTAL SODIUM (℞). Ampules. Amobarbital sodium. Dosages (intravenous) range from 65 to 500 mg. for children 6 to 12 years of age. Safety and effectiveness have not been established for children less than 6 years of age. The manufacturer makes no recommendations concerning children's doses for Amytal elixir and tablets.

√ *BUTICAPS* (℞). Capsules. Sodium butabarbital. Dosages for insomnia and daytime sedation depend on age, weight, and condition, as determined by your doctor. The dosage range for daytime sedation is 7.5 to 30 mg.

√ *BUTISOL SODIUM* (℞). Elixir. See BUTICAPS above.

NEMBUTAL (℞). Elixir. Pentobarbital. May be used to treat insomnia, but it is more often used for daytime sedation, convulsive conditions, and as a preoperative medication. Dosages for insomnia for all uses depend on age, weight, and condition as determined by your doctor.

NEMBUTAL SODIUM (℞). See NEMBUTAL above.

√ *PHENOBARBITAL* (℞). Capsules, drops, elixir. Phenobarbital. Dosages for insomnia depend on age, weight, and condition, as determined by your doctor. This drug is also used for daytime sedation, convulsive conditions, and as a pre- and postoperative medication.

√ *PHENOBARBITAL SODIUM* (℞). Ampules, vials, syringes, cartridge-needle units. Phenobarbital sodium. See PHENO-BARBITAL above.

SECONAL Elixir (℞). Secobarbital. Manufacturer's recommended doses are 50 to 100 mg., although safety and effectiveness in children have not been established.

SECONAL SODIUM (℞). Capsules, vials, suppositories. See SECONAL.

√ *SK-PHENOBARBITAL* (℞). Tablets. See PHENOBARBITAL in this section.

√ *SOLFOTON* (℞). Tablets, capsules, and sugar-coated (S/C) tablets. Phenobarbital. This drug is used to obtain sedation (day and night) over a long period. Dosage recommended by the manufacturer is 16 mg. every 6 hours, with no specific reference to children. Consult your doctor.

II. NONBARBITURATES

Trade name
   √ *DALMANE* (℞).

Ingredient
   Flurazepam, a member of the benzodiazepine family of drugs which includes Valium and Librium.

This drug is used to
   Induce sleep at bedtime and treat sleeplessness or interrupted sleep in children over 15 years of age. It is also used for pre- and postoperative sedation.

How this drug works
   The exact mechanism has not been established.

The FDA has
   ☑ Approved this drug.
   ☐ Not approved this drug.

This drug is
   ☑ Effective.*
   ☐ Probably effective.
   ☐ Ineffective.

*But not immediately. It may take about 2 to 3 days before this drug begins to work.

229

This drug should not be used under the following condition
- Sensitivity to flurazepam.

Your doctor may not approve use of this drug under the following conditions
- Severe mental depression.
- Liver or kidney disorders.

Use of the following drugs decreases the effectiveness of this drug
No drugs with this action reported.

How this drug interacts with other drugs
- Acts like barbiturates on other CNS depressants, including barbiturates. See page 225.
- Dalmane also reacts with other drugs less likely to be prescribed by your doctor. Inform your doctor of all drugs your child is taking. While your child is on Dalmane, do not give the child any other drug, prescription or nonprescription, without the approval of your doctor.

How this drug is supplied
Capsules.

Dosage
Your doctor will individualize dosage for children over 15 years of age.

Common side effects
Drowsiness, light-headedness, dizziness, slurred speech, unsteadiness, blurred vision, fatigue, constipation or diarrhea, stomach pain, difficulty in urinating, nausea, vomiting. *Warning:* This drug taken at bedtime may decrease alertness the following day. Should this side effect

occur, keep children from using machines, driving, or engaging in other potentially hazardous activities requiring alertness.

Effect of long-term use
    Possibly addictive.

After-use effects
    For a time, your child may experience nausea, vomiting, stomach cramps, sweating, trembling, irritability, nervousness, trouble sleeping, and convulsions or seizures.

Trade name
    √ *NOCTEC* (R).

Ingredient
    Chloral hydrate.

This drug is used to
    Induce sleep at bedtime and treat sleeplessness or interrupted sleep.

How this drug works
    The exact mechanism has not been established.

The FDA has
        ☑ Approved this drug.
        ☐ Not approved this drug.

This drug is
        ☑ Effective.*
        ☐ Probably effective.
        ☐ Ineffective.

This drug should not be used under the following conditions
    • Sensitivity to chloral hydrate.
    • Severe liver, kidney, or heart disorders.

Your doctor may not approve use of this drug under the following conditions
    • Heart disease.
    • Gastritis or stomach inflammation.

*Effectiveness may be lost after about 2 weeks of continued use.

232

Use of the following drugs decreases the effect of this drug
   No drugs with this action reported.

How this drug interacts with other drugs
   • Acts like barbiturates on CNS depressants, including barbiturates. See page 225.
   • Decreases the effectiveness of anticoagulants (blood thinners).
   • Noctec also reacts with other drugs less likely to be prescribed by your doctor. Inform your doctor of all drugs your child is taking. While your child is on Noctec, do not give the child any other drugs, prescription or nonprescription, without the approval of your doctor.

How this drug is supplied
   Capsules, syrup.

Dosage
   For insomnia, 50 mg. per kilogram (about 2.2 lb.) of body weight, in 1 or 2 doses, but never more than 1,000 mg.

Common side effects
   Nausea, vomiting, diarrhea, stomach irritation, skin rashes, hives, unsteadiness, dizziness.

Effect of long-term use
   Possibly addictive.

After-use effect
   Delirium may result following sudden withdrawal after use for a long period.

Trade name
NOLUDAR (℞).

Ingredient
Methyprylon.

This drug is used to
Induce sleep at bedtime for children over 12 years of age.

How this drug works
The exact mechanism has not been established.

The FDA has
☑ Approved this drug.
☐ Not approved this drug.

This drug is
☑ Effective.*
☐ Probably effective.
☐ Ineffective.

This drug should not be used under the following condition
• Sensitivity to methyprylon.

Your doctor may not approve use of this drug under the following conditions
• Liver or kidney disorders.
• Porphyria (a congenital nerve and muscle disease which may produce mental disorders).

*Effectiveness may be lost after about 1 week of continued use.

Use of the following drugs decreases the effectiveness of this drug
    No drugs with this action reported.

How this drug interacts with other drugs
- Acts like barbiturates on CNS depressants, including barbiturates. See page 225.
- Noludar also reacts with other drugs less likely to be prescribed by your doctor. Inform your doctor of all drugs your child is taking. While your child is on Noludar, do not give the child any other drug, prescription or nonprescription, without the approval of your doctor.

How this drug is supplied.
    Tablets.

Dosage
    At bedtime, 50 to 200 mg., as determined by your doctor.

Common side effects
    Dizziness, daytime drowsiness, headache, diarrhea, vomiting, rash, inflammation of the esophagus, low white blood cell count in circulating blood. *Warning:* This drug taken at bedtime may decrease alertness the following day. Should this side effect occur, keep children from using machines, driving, or engaging in other potentially hazardous activities requiring alertness.

Effect of long-term use
    Possibly addictive.

After-use effects
    Similar to those of barbiturates. See page 226.

DRUGS TO TREAT BED-WETTING

IMIPRAMINES

Trade names
    See page 238.

Ingredient
    Imipramine hydrochloride, a member of the tricyclic antidepressant family of drugs.

These drugs are used to
    Treat bed-wetting (enuresis) not caused by a physical disorder.

How these drugs work
    The exact mechanism has not been established. Imipramines have a moderate sedative action.

The FDA has
        ☑ Approved these drugs.
        ☐ Not approved these drugs.

These drugs are
        ☑ Effective.*
        ☐ Probably effective.
        ☐ Ineffective.

*Dosage of imipramine hydrochloride tablets may be increased if satisfactory response is not obtained after 1 week.

These drugs should not be used under the following conditions
- Sensitivity to this drug or chemically related drugs.
- During recovery from heart attack.

Your doctor may not approve use of these drugs under the following conditions
- Heart disease.
- High blood pressure.
- Asthma.
- Liver disease.
- Gastrointestinal problems.
- Manic-depressive psychosis.
- Schizophrenia.
- Epilepsy or other convulsive disorders.
- Kidney impairment.
- Thyroid disease.
- Glaucoma.

Use of the following drugs decreases the effectiveness of these drugs
No drugs with this action reported.

How these drugs interact with other drugs
- Act like barbiturates on other CNS depressants, including barbiturates. See page 225.
- Adverse reactions are possible when these drugs are used simultaneously with medicines for pain, allergies (including hay fever), colds, blood pressure, seizures, insomnia, thyroid conditions, sedation, and depression. Some of these reactions could be serious.
- Imipramines also react with other drugs less likely to be prescribed by your doctor. Inform your doctor of all drugs your child is taking. While your child is on imipramines, do not give the child any other drug,

prescription or nonprescription, without the approval of your doctor.

How these drugs are supplied
Tablets, capsules, vials.

Dosage
See individual drugs, beginning below.

Common side effects
Mild stomach upsets, drowsiness, nervousness, sleeping problems. These are likely to disappear as drug use continues.

Effects of long-term use
Adverse side effects other than those listed in the preceding paragraph may appear. Consult your doctor. Safety for long-term use has not been established.

After-use effects
Effects may persist from 3 to 7 days after termination.

The drugs
Imipramines are listed alphabetically by product name. The ingredient of each product is given, as well as dosage and other pertinent information not covered in the general description.

√ *IMIPRAMINE HCL TABLETS* (℞). Imipramine hydrochloride. Dosage for children over 6 years of age is 25 mg. 1 hour before bedtime. If response is unsatisfactory, dosage may be increased to 50 mg. for children up to 12 years of age, and 75 mg. for children over 12 years of age.

√ *JANIMINE FILMTAB TABLETS* (℞). Imipramine hydro-chloride. See IMIPRAMINE HCL TABLETS in this section.

√ *SK-PRAMINE*™ (℞). Tablets. Imipramine hydrochloride. See IMIPRAMINE HCL TABLETS in this section.

√ *TOFRANIL* (℞). Tablets, ampules. Imapramine hydro-chloride. Dosage: See IMIPRAMINE HCL TABLETS in this section. By injection (intramuscular only). Use is not recommended for children up to 12 years of age. *Caution:* Tofranil-PM, imapramine pamoate, is not recommended for children.

13

Rapid Guide to Miscellaneous Prescription Drugs for Children

The following list, arranged alphabetically by trade name, tells you at a glance what each drug is used for and, by referring to the MEANING OF THE CODE NUMBERS (see page 257), the status of the drug in relation to its use for children.

Drug Trade Name	This Drug Is Used for	Code
ABBOKINASE	Clotting disorders	2
ABSORBO CARPINE	Glaucoma	1
ADAPIN	Emotional/brain disorders	6
ADRUCIL	Cancer	1
A-HYDROCORT	Corticosteroid therapy	13, 37
AKINETON	Parkinson's disease	1
ALDACTAZIDE	Diuretic therapy	1
ALDOCLOR	Hypertension	1
ALDORIL	Hypertension	1
ALKERAN	Cancer	1
ALPHADERM	Dermatitis	1
ANAPROX	Mild/moderate pain	2
ANCOBAN	Fungal infections	1
ANDRIAMYCIN	Cancer	1

Drug Trade Name	This Drug Is Used for	Code
ANDROID	Male sexual hormone therapy	12, 13
ANTIVERT	Nausea and vomiting	5
ANTURANE	Gout	1
ANUSOL-HC	Hemorrhoids	10
APPRESAZIDE	Hypertension	1
APRESOLINE	Hypertension	1
ARISTOCORT	Corticosteroid therapy	13, 37
ARLIDEN	Peripheral circulatory disorders	1
ARTANE	Parkinson's disease	1
ARTHROMBIN-K	Clotting disorders	1
ASENDIN	Emotional/brain disorders	28
ATIVAN	Emotional/brain disorders	9, 17
ATROMID-5	High cholesterol/lipids	2
A/T/S	Acne	1
AVC	Fungal infections	1
AZO GANTANOL	Antibiotic therapy	6
AZOGANTROSIN	Antibiotic therapy	6
BEEF LEUTE ILETIN	Diabetes	1
BEEF NPH ILETIN	Diabetes	1
BEEF PROTAMIN ZINC AND ILETIN	Diabetes	1
BEEF REGULAR ILETIN	Diabetes	1
BELLERGAL/ BELLERGAL-S	Ulcers/GI disorders	1
BENDECTIN	Nausea and vomiting	8
BENZAC	Acne	1
BENZAC W	Acne	1
BICNU	Cancer	1
BIPHETAMINE	Appetite suppression	6

Drug Trade Name	This Drug Is Used for	Code
BLENOXANE	Cancer	1
BLEPH-10	Eye infections	1
BRETYLOL	Cardiac arrhythmias	2
BRONKOSOL	Asthma	1
BRONKOULETER	Asthma	1
BUTAZOLIDIN	Arthritis	18
BUTAZOLIDIN-ALKA	Arthritis	18
CAFERGOT	Headaches	1
CAFERGOT P-B	Headaches	1
CALCIPARINE	Clotting disorders	1
CARBACEL	Glaucoma	1
CARDILATE	Angina pectoris	1
CATAPRES	Hypertension	2
CELESTONE	Corticosteroid therapy	13, 37
CELESTONE PHOSPHATE	Corticosteroid therapy	13, 37
CELESTONE SOLUSPAN	Corticosteroid therapy	13, 37
CENTRAX	Emotional/brain disorders	19, 24
CERUBIDINE	Cancer	5
CETACORT	Dermatitis	1
CHLOROPTIC	Eye infections	1
CHRONULAC	Constipation	1
CLEOCIN T	Acne	1
CLINORAL	Arthritis	1
COGENTIN	Parkinson's disease	1
COL BENEMID	Gout	35, 36
COLCHICINE	Gout	1
COMBID	Ulcers/GI disorders	6
COMBIPRES	Hypertension	2
CORDRAN	Dermatitis	1
CORDRAN-N	Dermatitis	1
CORDRAN-SP	Dermatitis	1

Drug Trade Name	This Drug Is Used for	Code
CORGARD	Angina pectoris, hypertension	2
CORT-DOME	Dermatitis	1
CORTEF	Corticosteroid therapy	13, 37
CORTEF ACETATE	Corticosteroid therapy	13, 37
CORTEF FLUID	Corticosteroid therapy	13, 37
CORTISONE ACETATE	Corticosteroid therapy	37
CORTISPORIN CREAM	Dermatitis	1
CORTISPORIN OINTMENT	Dermatitis	1
COUMADIN	Clotting disorders	1
CURRETAB	Female sexual hormone therapy	1
CYCLOCORT	Dermatitis	1
CYCLOSPASMOL	Peripheral circulatory disorders	1
CYTOXIN	Cancer	1
DALMANE	Sleeping disorders	31
DARANIDE	Glaucoma	1
DARVOCET-N 50/N100	Mild/moderate pain	5
DARVON	Mild/moderate pain	5
DARVON-N	Mild/moderate pain	5
DECADERM	Dermatitis	1
DECADRON	Corticosteroid therapy	13, 37
DECADRON LA-SUSPENSION	Corticosteroid therapy	37, 38
DECADRON PHOSPHATE	Corticosteroid therapy	13, 37
DELATESTRYL	Male sexual hormone therapy	14
DELTASONE	Corticosteroid therapy	13, 37
DEPO-MEDROL	Corticosteroid therapy	13, 37

Drug Trade Name	This Drug Is Used for	Code
DEPO-PROVERA	Female sexual hormone therapy	1
DEPO-TESTOSTERONE	Male sexual hormone therapy	14
DESQUAM-X5	Acne	1
DESQUAM-X10	Acne	1
DESQUAM X WASH	Acne	1
DIABESE	Diabetes	11
DIAMOX	Glaucoma	1
DIDREX	Appetite suppression	6
DIETHYLSTILBESTROL	Female sexual hormone therapy	13, 15
DILAUDID	Strong pain relief	2
DILAUDID COUGH SYRUP	Coughs	2
DIPROSONE	Dermatitis	1
DIULO	Diuretic therapy	5
DIUPRES	Hypertension	1
DIURIL INTRAVENOUS SODIUM	Diuretic therapy	5
DOPAR	Parkinson's disease	1
DORIDEN	Sleeping disorders	5
DUO-MEDIHALER	Asthma	1
DURACEF	Antibiotic therapy	3
DYAZIDE	Diuretic therapy	1, 3
DYMELOR	Diabetes	11
DYRENIUM	Congestive heart failure	1
E-CARPINE	Glaucoma	1
ECONOCHLOR	Eye infections	1
ELAVIL	Emotional/brain disorders	6
EMETE-CON	Nausea and vomiting	5
EMPERIN WITH CODEINE	Mild/moderate pain	1

Drug Trade Name	This Drug Is Used for	Code
ENDEP	Emotional/brain disorders	6
ENDURON	Diuretic therapy	1
ENDURONYL	Hypertension	1
ENDURONYL/FORTE	Hypertension	1
EPIFRIN	Glaucoma	2
E-PILO	Glaucoma	1
EQUAGESIC	Musculoskeletal pain	6
ERGOSTAT	Headaches	1
ESKALITH	Emotional/brain disorders	5
ESKATROL	Appetite suppression	6
ESMIL	Hypertension	1
ESTRACE	Female sexual hormone therapy	13, 15
ESTROVIS	Female sexual hormone therapy	13, 15
FASTIN	Appetite suppression	6
FIORINAL	Headaches	9
FIORINAL WITH CODEINE	Mild/moderate pain	1
FLEXERIL	Musculoskeletal pain	20
FLORONE	Dermatitis	1
FLUOROURCIL	Cancer	1
FUNGIZONE	Fungal infections	1
GANTRISIN OPHTHALMIC	Eye infections	1
GEOCILLIN	Antibiotic therapy	1
GLOBIN ZINC INSULIN	Diabetes	1
GLOBIN ZINC INSULIN (beef and pork pancreas)	Diabetes	1
GYNE-LOTRIMIN	Fungal infections	1
GYNERGEN	Headaches	1

Drug Trade Name	This Drug Is Used for	Code
HALDOL	Emotional/brain disorders	29, 30
HALOG	Dermatitis	1
HALOTESTIN	Female sexual hormone therapy	14
HALOTEX	Fungal infections	1
HEPARIN SODIUM	Clotting disorders	1
HYCOMINE	Coughs/colds	1
HYDERGINE	Peripheral circulatory disorders	1
HYDROCORTONE	Corticosteroid therapy	13, 37
HYDROPRES	Hypertension	1
HYGROTON	Diuretic therapy	1
HYTONE	Dermatitis	1
ILOTYCIN OPHTHALMIC	Eye infections	1
IMODIUM	Diarrhea	6
INDERAL	Angina pectoris, cardiac arrythmias, migraine, hypertension	3
INDERIDE	Hypertension	1
INDOCIN	Arthritis	32, 33
INSULIN	Diabetes	1
INSULIN ZINC SUSPENSION	Diabetes	1
INSULIN ZINC SUSPENSION, EXTENDED	Diabetes	1
INSULIN ZINC SUSPENSION, PROMPT	Diabetes	1
IOMANIN	Appetite suppression	6
ISMELIN	Hypertension	1
ISOPHANE INSULIN	Diabetes	1
ISOPHANE INSULIN SUSPENSION	Diabetes	1

Drug Trade Name	This Drug Is Used for	Code
ISOPTO-CARBACHOL	Glaucoma	1
ISOPTO CARBINE	Glaucoma	1
ISORDAL	Angina pectoris	1
KAOCHLOR	Potassium supplementation	1
KAOCHLOR-EFF	Potassium supplementation	1
KAOCHLOR-SF	Potassium supplementation	1
KAON-CL TABS	Potassium supplementation	1
KAON ELIXIR	Potassium supplementation	1
KAY CIEL	Potassium supplementation	1
KEMADRIN	Parkinson's disease	1
KENACORT	Corticosteroid therapy	13, 37
KENALOG	Corticosteroid therapy, dermatitis	13, 37, 1
KENALOG-H	Dermatitis	1
K-LOR	Potassium supplementation	1
KLORVESS	Potassium supplementation	1
KLOTRIX	Potassium supplementation	1
K-LYTE	Potassium supplementation	1
K-LYTE/DS	Potassium supplementation	1
LARODOPA	Parkinson's disease	1
LEUKERAN	Cancer	1

Drug Trade Name	This Drug Is Used for	Code
LEUTE ILETIN	Diabetes	1
LEUTE INSULIN	Diabetes	1
LIBRAX	Ulcers/GI disorders	1
LIDEX	Dermatitis	1
LIDEX-E	Dermatitis	1
LIMBITROL	Emotional/brain disorders	9, 17
LIORESAL	Musculoskeletal pain	6
LITHIUM CARBONATE	Emotional/brain disorders	5
LITHIUM CITRATE	Emotional/brain disorders	5
LOPRESSOR	Hypertension	2
LORELCO	High cholesterol/lipids	2
LOTRIMIN	Fungal infections	1
LOXITANE	Emotional/brain disorders	7
LOXITANE-C	Emotional/brain disorders	7
LOXITANE-IM	Emotional/brain disorders	7
LUDIOMIL	Emotional/brain disorders	19
LUFYLLIN	Asthma	1
MAOLATE	Musculoskeletal pain	6
MARPLAN	Emotional/brain disorders	7
MECLOMEN	Arthritis	35
MEDIHALER-ISO	Asthma	1
MEDROL	Corticosteroid therapy	13, 37
MEGACE	Cancer	1
MEQUIN	Sleeping disorders	5
METANDREN	Male sexual hormone therapy	12, 13
METHOTREXATE	Cancer	1
METICORTEN	Corticosteroid therapy	13, 37
MICATIN	Fungal infections	1
MICRAININ	Mild/moderate pain	6
MIDRIN	Headaches	1
MIGRAL	Headaches	1

Drug Trade Name	This Drug Is Used for	Code
MINIPRESS	Hypertension	2
MINIZIDE	Hypertension	2
MONISTAT 7	Fungal infections	1
MOTRIN	Mild/moderate pain, arthritis	2
MUCOMYST	Asthma	1
MUTAMYCIN	Cancer	1
MYCELEX	Fungal infections	1
MYCELEX-G	Fungal infections	1
MYCELEX-6	Fungal infections	1
MYCOLOG	Dermatitis	1
NALFON	Arthritis	2
NALFON 200	Mild/moderate pain	2
NAPROSYN	Arthritis, mild/moderate pain	2
NARDIL	Emotional/brain disorders	7
NAVANE	Emotional/brain disorders	2, 6
NEOSPORIN OPHTHALMIC OINTMENT	Eye infections	1
NEOSPORIN OPHTHALMIC SOLUTION	Eye infections	1
NEO-SYNALAR	Dermatitis	1
NICOTINIC ACID	High cholesterol/lipids	4
NITRO-BID	Angina pectoris	1
NITRO-STAT	Angina pectoris	1
NOLVADEX	Cancer	8
NORGESIC	Muscoskeletal pain	2, 6
NORPACE	Cardiac arrhythmias	2
NORPRAMIN	Emotional/brain disorders	5
NPH ILETIN	Diabetes	1

Drug Trade Name	This Drug Is Used for	Code
OGEN	Female sexual hormone therapy	13, 15
OPTIMINE	Allergies	6
ORASONE	Corticosteroid therapy	13, 37
ORETON METHYL	Male sexual hormone therapy	12, 13
ORINASE	Diabetes	11
ORTHO DIENESTROL CREAM	Female sexual hormone therapy	13, 15
OTK-DOME	Cancer	1
P1E1	Glaucoma	1
P2E1	Glaucoma	1
P3E1	Glaucoma	1
P6E1	Glaucoma	1
PAMELOR	Emotional/brain disorders	5
PAN OXYL	Acne	1
PAN OXYL AG	Acne	1
PANWARFIN	Clotting disorders	1
PARAFON FORTE	Male sexual hormone therapy	1
PARNATE	Emotional/brain disorders	1
PATHIBAMATE	Ulcers/GI disorders	6
PAVABID	Peripheral circulatory disorders	1
PERCOCET-5	Strong pain	5
PERITRATE	Angina pectoris	1
PERITRATE/SA	Angina pectoris	1
PERSA-GEL	Acne	1
PERSANTINE	Angina pectoris	1
PERTOFRANE	Emotional/brain disorders	5
PHENERGAN EXPEC-TORANT PLAIN	Coughs/colds	1

Drug Trade Name	This Drug Is Used for	Code

PHENERGAN EXPEC-
  TORANT WITH
  CODEINE
	Coughs	13

PILOCAR	Glaucoma	1
PILOCEL	Glaucoma	1
PLACIDYL	Sleeping disorders	5
PLATINOL	Cancer	1
POLYSPORIN OPHTHALMIC	Eye infections	1
PONSTEL	Mild/moderate pain	18
PORK LEUTE ILETIN II	Diabetes	1
PORK NPH ILETIN II	Diabetes	1
PORK PROTAMIN, ZINC AND ILETIN II	Diabetes	1
PORK REGULAR ILETIN	Diabetes	1
PREDNISOLONE	Corticosteroid therapy	13, 37
PRELUDIN	Appetite suppression	6
PREMARIN	Female sexual hormone therapy	13, 15

PREMARIN VAGINAL
  CREAM
	Female sexual hormone
	  therapy
		13, 15

PRO-BANTHINE	Ulcers/GI disorders	3
PROCAN SR	Cardiac arrhythmias	2
PROLOID	Thyroid disorders	1
PROLOPRIM	Antibiotic therapy	16, 17
PRONESTYL	Cardiac arrhythmias	1
PROSTIGMIN	Myasthenia gravis	1
PROTAMIN ZINC INSULIN	Diabetes	1
PROTOFOAM-HC	Hemorrhoids	1
PROVERA	Females sexual hormone therapy	1
PROXILIN	Emotional/brain disorders	2,6
P.V. CARPINE	Glaucoma	1

Drug Trade Name	This Drug Is Used for	Code
QUESTRIN	High cholesterol/lipids	1
QUINAGLUTE	Cardiac arrhythmias	1
QUINAMIN	Male sexual hormone therapy	1
QUINIDEX	Cardiac arrhythmias	1
RAUZIDE	Hypertension	1
REGROTON	Hypertension	1
REGULAR CONCEN-TRATED ILETIN	Diabetes	1
REGULAR ILETIN	Diabetes	1
RENOQUID	Antibiotic therapy	18
RETIN A	Acne	1
ROBAXIN	Musculoskeletal pain	9, 17, 21
ROBAXISAL	Musculoskeletal pain	2
RU-VERT	Nausea and vomiting	1
SALUTENSIN	Hypertension	1
SANOREX	Appetite suppression	6
SANSERT	Headaches	5
S-BENZAGEL	Acne	1
SEMILEUTE ILETIN	Diabetes	1
SER-AP-ES	Hypertension	1
SERAX	Emotional/brain disorders	25, 26
SERENTIL	Emotional/brain disorders	3, 6
SERPASIL	Hypertension	1
SINEMET	Parkinson's disease	19
SINEQUAN	Emotional/brain disorders	6
SINGLET	Colds	6
SKELAXIN	Musculoskeletal pain	2
SLOW-K	Potassium supplementation	1

Drug Trade Name	This Drug Is Used for	Code
SODIUM SULAMYD	Eye infections	1
SOLU-CORTEF	Corticosteroid therapy	13, 37
SOMA	Musculoskeletal pain	6
SOMA COMPOUND	Musculoskeletal pain	22,23
SOMA COMPOUND WITH CODEINE	Musculoskeletal pain	22, 23
SORBITRATE	Angina pectoris	1
STOXIL	Eye infections	1
STREPTASE	Clotting disorders	2
SURMONTIL	Emotional/brain disorders	5
SYNALAR	Dermatitis	1
SYNALAR-HP	Dermatitis	1, 35
SYNALOG-DC	Strong pain	2
SYNEMOL	Dermatitis	35
TACE	Female sexual hormone therapy	13, 15
TAGAMET	Ulcers/GI disorders	7
TALWIN 50	Strong pain	6
TANDEARIL	Arthritis	18
10-BENZAGELD 1	Acne	1
TENUATE	Appetite suppression	6
TEPANIL	Appetite suppression	6
TERPIN HYDRATE WITH CODEINE ELIXIR	Coughs	1
TESTRED	Male sexual hormone therapy	12, 13
THIOTEPA	Cancer	1
TIMOPTIC	Glaucoma	5
T-IONATE-PA	Male sexual hormone therapy	14
TOFRANIL-PM	Emotional/brain disorders	5
TOLINASE	Diabetes	11

Drug Trade Name	This Drug Is Used for	Code
TOPICORT	Dermatitis	1
TOPICYCLINE	Acne	1
TORECAN	Nausea and vomiting	9
TRAFON	Emotional/brain disorders	5
TRANXENE	Emotional/brain disorders	27
TRIAVIL	Emotional/brain disorders	5
TRILAFON	Emotional/brain disorders	6
TRIMPEX	Antibiotic therapy	16, 17
TRISILATE	Arthritis	5
TYLOX	Strong pain	5
ULTRALEUTE ILETIN	Diabetes	1
ULTRALEUTE INSULIN	Diabetes	1
URIPAS	Urinary incontinence	5
VAGISEC PLUS	Fungal infections	1
VAGITROL	Fungal infections	1
VALISONE	Dermatitis	1
VANOBID	Fungal infections	7
VASODILAN	Peripheral circulatory disorders	1
VERSTRAN	Emotional/brain disorders	19, 24
VICODIN	Strong pain	6
VIOFORM	Dermatitis	1
VIRA-A OPHTHALMIC OINTMENT	Eye infections	1
VOSOL HC OTIC SOLUTION	Ear infections	1
VOSOL OTIC SOLUTION	Ear infections	1
VOXIN-PG	Respiratory disorders	6

Drug Trade Name	This Drug Is Used for	Code
WIGRAINE	Headaches	1
WORFLEX	Musculoskeletal pain	6
WYGESIC	Mild/moderate pain	5
XYLOCAINE	Cardiac arrhythmias	1
ZAROXOLYN	Diuretic therapy	5

MEANING OF THE CODE NUMBERS

(Refers to use by children only)

1. No guidelines set.
2. No definite proof of safety and effectiveness.
3. No definite proof of safety.
4. No definite proof of safety and effectiveness in large doses.
5. Do not use.
6. Do not use in children less than 12 years old.
7. Do not use in children less than 16 years old unless possible advantages outweigh possible adverse reactions.
8. Not useful to children.
9. No definite proof of safety in children under 12 years old.
10. Use with caution.
11. Do not use in juvenile or growth-onset diabetes.
12. Use cautiously in young boys.
13. Dosages not set.
14. Do not use in boys prior to puberty.
15. Use cautiously in growing children.
16. No definite proof of safety in children less than 2 months old.
17. No definite proof of effectiveness in children under 12 years old.
18. Do not use in children less than 14 years old.
19. No definite proof of safety in children less than 18 years old.

20. No proof of safety and effectiveness in children less than 15 years old.
21. May be used in case of tetanus.
22. Do not use in children less than 5 years old.
23. No guidelines set for children less than 5 years old.
24. No definite proof of effectiveness in children less than 18 years old.
25. Do not use in children less than 6 years old.
26. No dosage guidelines for children between 6 and 12 years old.
27. Do not use in children less than 18 years old.
28. No definite proof of safety and effectiveness in children less than 16 years old.
29. No guidelines set for oral dosage.
30. Do not use in other than oral form.
31. Do not use in children less than 15 years old.
32. Do not use in children less than 14 years old unless other drugs are unsuitable.
33. Careful medical monitoring is mandatory.
34. No definite proof of safety and effectiveness in children less than 14 years old.
35. Do not use in children less than 2 years old.
36. No guidelines set for children more than 2 years old.
37. Medical monitoring of growth and development is mandatory in extended treatment.
38. No dosage guidelines set for children less than 12 years old.

Index